Healthy Living Tips

Unlock the Path to Wellness: Expert Healthy Living Tips for a Vibrant Life

Thomas T. Stewart

Table content

CONTENT 1

INTRODUCTION

Carrying on with a solid way of life isn't simply a brief pattern; a groundbreaking excursion enables people to embrace their maximum capacity. This segment will establish the groundwork until the end of the aide by presenting the idea of sound living and its importance in our lives.

1.1 Understanding Healthy Living. Healthy living is a multifaceted strategy that takes into account one's mental, emotional, and physical health. It goes beyond merely exercising occasionally or eating a restrictive diet. It includes settling on cognizant decisions that help generally wellbeing and essentialness. By understanding the multi-layered parts of sound living, people can accomplish enduring enhancements in their personal satisfaction.

1.2 The Importance of a Balanced Diet. The foundation of a healthy lifestyle is a well-balanced diet. Consuming a wide range of nutrient-dense foods, such as fruits, vegetables, whole grains, lean proteins, and healthy fats, is necessary for this to happen. This segment will dive into the advantages of every nutrition type, featuring the fundamental nutrients and minerals they give, and how they add to our prosperity.

1.3 Consolidating Normal Exercise

Active work is a vital part of solid living. Regular exercise not only boosts mood and cognitive function but also strengthens muscles and improves cardiovascular health. This part will investigate different types of activity, from cardiovascular exercises to strength preparing and adaptability works out, while stressing the significance of finding exercises that give pleasure and satisfaction.

1.4 Stress Management and Mental Health In today's fast-paced world, stress has become a common health problem. This segment will reveal insight into the effect of weight on both physical and emotional well-being. After that, it will talk about effective ways to deal with stress, like practicing mindfulness, relaxing, and developing a positive attitude.

Stressing the association between the psyche and body, the aide will highlight how a sound mental state is fundamental for by and large prosperity.

Through this thorough presentation, perusers will acquire a reasonable comprehension of the expansive extent of sound living and how every perspective adds to an agreeable and flourishing presence. In the following chapters, readers will learn more about specific topics and receive expert guidance and practical suggestions to help them achieve a healthier and happier life.

Figuring out Sound Living: Embrace the Way to Deep rooted Wellness

Solid living isn't simply a transitory prevailing fashion or an accident diet; a strong and persevering through way of life opens the potential for a satisfying and energetic presence. At its center, sound living is a comprehensive methodology that envelops each part of our being - from actual wellness to mental prosperity, from feeding our bodies to developing significant connections. We should leave on an excursion to investigate the complexities of solid living and uncover the key to accomplishing long haul prosperity.

The Comprehensive Idea of Sound Living

Solid living rises above simple actual wellbeing. It perceives the interconnectedness of our physical, mental, and profound viewpoints. Similarly as a reasonable biological system flourishes when every one of its parts are as one, so does our prosperity when we encourage balance inside ourselves. By sustaining every feature, we make a positive expanding influence that spreads to all parts of our lives.

1. Nutrition for the Body. Consuming wholesome, nutrient-dense foods is an essential component of maintaining a healthy lifestyle. The food we eat is the fuel that empowers us and generally supports physical processes. We get the essential nutrients we need to perform at our best when we eat a well-balanced diet full of fruits, vegetables, whole grains, lean proteins, and healthy fats.

2. Strategies for an Active Lifestyle. Movement is the essence of life, and physical activity is the key to realizing our potential. Taking part in standard activity upgrades our actual wellbeing as well as cultivates mental clearness and profound prosperity. Finding exercises that impact us permits us to find bliss in development, changing activity from an errand to a wellspring of delight.

3. Supporting Mental and Close to home Well-Being

A sound psyche is the underpinning of a sound body. Really focusing on our emotional well-being includes embracing rehearses like care, contemplation, and stress the board strategies. We equip ourselves to face life's challenges with grace and poise by cultivating emotional intelligence and resilience.

4. Quality Rest and Rest

In our speedy world, the value of rest is frequently underrated. However, sleep is essential to rejuvenation because it allows our minds and bodies to heal and regenerate. We can expect to wake up feeling rejuvenated and ready to tackle each day with vigor if we put sound sleep habits first.

5. Building Strong Relationships. Human connection is an essential need. Our souls are nourished and supported by meaningful relationships during both good times and bad. Our lives are profoundly enhanced by healthy relationships, which foster growth, empathy, and comprehension.

6. Striking a Balance. To live a long and healthy life, it is essential to strike a balance between work, leisure, and personal time. We can avoid burnout and keep our daily sense of fulfillment by balancing our commitments.

Conclusion: Recognizing the importance of maintaining a healthy lifestyle is the first step toward a life filled with joy, vitality, and contentment. We give ourselves the ability to thrive in every sphere of our being by embracing the holistic nature of this way of life. As we leave on this excursion together, let us open the potential inside ourselves and set out on a way towards deep rooted health. Are you prepared to begin the process? How about we start!

CONTENT 2

Knowledge of Healthy Living: Embrace the Way to Deep rooted Wellness

Solid living isn't simply a transitory craze or an accident diet; a strong and getting through way of life opens the potential for a satisfying and lively presence. Healthy living is, at its core, a holistic approach that encompasses all aspects of our being, including physical fitness, mental health, body nutrition, and meaningful relationships. Let's set out on a journey to learn about the intricacies of living a healthy lifestyle and the ways to achieve long-term happiness.

The All encompassing Nature of Sound Living

Sound living rises above simple actual wellbeing. It perceives the interconnectedness of our physical, mental, and profound viewpoints. Our well-being improves when we cultivate internal harmony, just as a balanced ecosystem does when all of its components function in harmony. We create a positive ripple effect that extends to all aspects of our lives by nurturing each aspect.

1. Supporting the Body

A foundation of solid living lies in supporting our bodies with healthy and supplement rich food sources. The food we devour is the fuel that invigorates us and generally supports physical processes. We get the essential nutrients we need to perform at our best when we eat a well-balanced diet full of fruits, vegetables, whole grains, lean proteins, and healthy fats.

2. Strategies for an Active Lifestyle. Movement is the essence of life, and physical activity is the key to realizing our potential. Regular exercise improves our mental clarity and emotional well-being in addition to our physical health. Finding exercises that impact us permits us to find euphoria in development, changing activity from an errand to a wellspring of delight.

3. Taking Care of One's Mental and Emotional Health. A healthy mind is the foundation of a healthy body. Really focusing on our emotional well-being includes embracing rehearses like care, reflection, and stress the executives strategies. By developing the ability to understand people at their core and versatility, we prepare ourselves to explore life's difficulties with effortlessness and balance.

4. Rest and Quality Sleep. In our fast-paced world, the significance of quality sleep is frequently undervalued. However, rest is the foundation of revival, permitting our bodies and psyches to recuperate and recover. Focusing on tranquil rest propensities guarantees we awaken invigorated and prepared to require on every day with force.

5. Cultivating Sound Relationships

Human association is a principal human need. Developing significant connections feeds our spirits and offers help during both delights and difficulties. Our lives are profoundly enhanced by healthy relationships, which foster growth, empathy, and comprehension.

6. Making progress toward Balance

Finding some kind of harmony between work, recreation, and individual time is imperative to manageable solid living. Adjusting responsibilities guarantees we stay balanced and keep a feeling of satisfaction in our regular routines.

Conclusion: Recognizing the importance of maintaining a healthy lifestyle is the first step toward a life filled with joy, vitality, and contentment. By embracing the comprehensive idea of this way of life, we enable ourselves to flourish in each part of our being. Let us unlock our potential and set out on a path toward long-term wellness as we embark on this journey together. Are you prepared to begin the process? Let's start!

2.1 The Value of a Healthy Diet: Support Your Body, Fuel Your Life

A reasonable eating regimen is the bedrock of a sound way of life, enabling us with the essential supplements to help our physical and mental prosperity. It goes beyond counting calories and following a strict diet; it's tied in with supporting our bodies with a different exhibit of food sources that give fundamental nutrients, minerals, and macronutrients. In this segment, we'll dive into the meaning of a fair eating regimen and investigate the advantages it offers for general wellbeing and imperativeness.

1 . A well-balanced diet ensures that our bodies receive all of the nutrients they require to function at their best. This incorporates macronutrients like sugars, proteins, and fats, which give energy and back important physical processes. It additionally incorporates micronutrients like nutrients and minerals, which are fundamental for different physiological cycles, like digestion, resistant capability, and bone wellbeing. We can avoid nutrient deficiencies and promote a healthy body by eating a variety of foods.

2. Maintaining Energy Levels . Our bodies use food as their primary energy source. A decent eating regimen

gives a consistent stockpile of energy over the course of the day, forestalling energy crashes and exhaustion. The blend of perplexing starches, lean proteins, and solid fats guarantees that we keep up with consistent glucose levels, advancing supported energy and mental sharpness.

3. Supporting Weight Management

Keeping a sound weight is vital for generally speaking prosperity. A fair eating regimen oversees weight by giving the right supplements while controlling calorie consumption. Food sources wealthy in fiber and protein add to sensations of completion, lessening the probability of gorging. Besides, a reasonable eating regimen empowers a sound connection with food, zeroing in on sustenance as opposed to limitation or hardship.

4. Improving Resistant Function

A very much fed body flaunts a strong invulnerable framework, fit for guarding against diseases and sicknesses. Supporting the immune system relies heavily on antioxidants, vitamins C and D, zinc, and other nutrients. A fair eating routine wealthy in natural products, vegetables, entire grains, and lean proteins fortifies our body's safeguards, assisting us with remaining better and stronger.

5. Promoting Heart Health

A healthy diet can have a significant impact on heart health by lowering the risk of heart disease. Diets high in unsaturated fats and low in saturated and trans fats support healthy cholesterol levels and cardiovascular health. Furthermore, integrating heart-quality food varieties like sleek fish, nuts, and entire grains can assist with keeping up with ideal circulatory strain and lessen the gamble of coronary illness.

6. Further developing Stomach related Health

Fiber-rich food sources, like natural products, vegetables, and entire grains, are fundamental for stomach related wellbeing. They advance ordinary solid discharges, forestall stoppage, and backing a sound stomach microbiome. A well-functioning digestive system, enhanced nutrient absorption, and overall gut health are all benefits of a well-balanced diet high in fiber.

Conclusion

Embracing a reasonable eating regimen is a crucial stage towards an energetic and flourishing life. By feeding our bodies with a different cluster of supplement rich food varieties, we support our actual prosperity, mental clearness, and close to home equilibrium. A plate of colorful fruits and vegetables, lean proteins, whole grains, and healthy fats—a symphony of flavors that gives you energy and vitality—should be your goal. Keep in mind that a healthy diet includes more than just what you eat today; it's tied in with developing economical dietary patterns that will help you into the indefinite future. Allow food to be your partner in the excursion towards ideal wellbeing and prosperity!

2.2 Including Regular Physical Activity: Open Your Body's True capacity, Embrace the Delight of Movement

In the domain of solid living, normal activity is the unique power that drives us towards an existence of essentialness, strength, and bliss. A long way past the bounds of a tedious exercise routine daily practice, practice is an elating excursion of self-disclosure and change. In this section, we'll explore the fascinating world of exercise and how it profoundly affects our mental health, physical health, and overall enthusiasm for life.

1. Developing Physical Strength and Endurance

Regular exercise is the key to unlocking our body's potential, developing strength, and enhancing endurance. Taking part in cardiovascular exercises like running, cycling, or swimming hoists our pulse, working on cardiovascular wellness and supporting lung limits. Strength preparing works out, then again, shape and tone our muscles, expanding practical strength and advancing bone thickness. Embrace the engaging sensation of being competent and versatile as your body adjusts and turns out to be stronger with every exercise.

2. Lifting Temperament and Profound Well-Being

Past its actual advantages, practice is a strong state of mind enhancer, delivering endorphins - the vibe great chemicals - that lift our spirits and decrease pressure. Whether it's an energetic stroll in nature or an empowering dance meeting, practice has the mind blowing capacity to dissolve away pressure, nervousness, and weariness, leaving us feeling restored and good. As you embark on a journey toward emotional well-being, take advantage of the cathartic release that exercise provides.

3. Developing Care and Present-Second Awareness

Practice offers a valuable chance to develop care, moving our concentration to the current second. Exercise encourages us to be fully present in the experience, freeing our minds from the chatter of everyday life, whether it's through the rhythmic motion of a yoga flow or the conscious coordination of a martial arts practice. Embrace the reflective nature of activity, appreciating every development and sensation as you discover an authentic sense of harmony in the midst of the movement.

4. Building Associations and Community

The quest for normal activity opens ways to a universe of shared interests and fellowship. Exercise fosters connections and community, whether in a gym class, a local sports team, or an outdoor fitness group. Embrace the help and support of similar people as you challenge each other to arrive at new levels and celebrate triumphs together.

5. Reducing the Risk of Chronic Disease

Regular physical activity is a powerful defense against chronic diseases like heart disease, type 2 diabetes, and some cancers. We can improve insulin sensitivity, maintain healthy blood pressure, and improve blood circulation by regularly exercising. Accept the fact that every workout is an investment in your health and well-being over the long term.

Conclusion. Adding regular exercise to your routine is a thrilling journey of personal development and self-discovery. It offers you the gift of a stronger body, a lighter spirit, and a deeper connection to yourself and others by transcending the confines of a routine. Embrace the delight of development, enjoy each step, and revel in the elation of stretching your boundaries. Allow exercise to be your dependable sidekick on this wondrous excursion towards an existence of limitless essentialness and enthusiasm. In this way, trim up those shoes, get that yoga mat, or jump on that bicycle - the experience anticipates, and the advantages are unimaginable!

2.3 Overseeing Pressure and Mental Prosperity: Releasing Internal Amicability, Embracing Serenity

In the clamoring ensemble of life, stress can frequently be an unwanted buddy, pulling at our souls and blurring our brains. However, inside the domain of sound living, lies a significant craftsmanship - the specialty of overseeing pressure and sustaining mental prosperity. In this part, we'll leave on an extraordinary excursion to find strong strategies that lead us towards inward congruence, permitting us to embrace serenity in the midst of life's difficulties.

1. Unwinding the Effect of Stress

Understanding pressure is the most vital move towards restraining its strong hold. Stress is a characteristic reaction to life's requests, however delayed or over the top pressure can negatively affect our psychological and actual wellbeing. It's essential to perceive the indications of stress, which might appear as uneasiness, peevishness, rest unsettling influences, or even actual side effects like migraines or muscle strain.

2. Practicing Mindfulness and Meditation

Mindfulness, the art of being completely present in the moment without judging, is one of the most effective strategies for stress management. Through care rehearses, like reflection, profound breathing, or body check works out, we figure out how to isolate from hustling contemplations and anchor ourselves in the present. Allowing your mind to find peace in the midst of life's turmoil is a gift that you should embrace.

3. The Force of Positive Thinking

Our contemplations have the unprecedented ability to shape our existence. By developing a positive mentality and rehearsing self-empathy, we can balance pressure and improve our versatility. Embrace the propensity for appreciation, enjoying life's little delights, and testing negative idea designs with certifications and useful self-talk.

4. Engaging in Creative Activities
 Engaging in creative activities can be a balm for the soul, a means of expressing one's emotions, and a way to find solace in the midst of chaos. Whether it's painting, composing, moving, or playing music, innovative exercises give a road to self-articulation, permitting us to handle feelings and restore our spirits.

5. Seeking Connection and Support
When stress is weighing us down, it can be extremely healing to seek connection and support. Trust in a confided in a companion, relative, or specialist to discuss your thoughts and encounters. Knowing that we are not alone in our struggles and that reaching out is a

brave act of self-care, embrace the strength of vulnerability.

6. The Endowment of Self-Care

Amidst life's requests, we mustn't fail to remember the endowment of taking care of oneself. Getting some margin to sustain ourselves through unwinding, side interests, or exercises we appreciate, is fundamental for keeping up with mental prosperity. Embrace the idea that taking care of oneself isn't narrow minded; it is a demonstration of recharging, permitting us to be at our best for us and others.

Conclusion

Overseeing pressure and supporting mental prosperity is a groundbreaking excursion of self-disclosure and development. By embracing care, positive reasoning, innovativeness, association, and taking care of oneself, we develop inward agreement and construct profound flexibility. As we cross the ups and downs of life's embroidery, let us recall that inside us lies the ability to embrace tranquility in the midst of the tempests and encourage a significant feeling of prosperity. Thus, take a full breath, enjoy the present, and leave on a journey of mental and profound investigation - an excursion towards a day to day existence improved with harmony, bliss, and happiness.

CONTENT 3

Taking Care of Your Body: The Craft of Culinary Wellbeing and Healthy Nutrition

In the lively embroidered artwork of solid living, feeding your body frames the lovely show-stopper that fills your existence with imperativeness and prosperity. Past the domain of simple food, sustenance incorporates a wonderful excursion of culinary wellbeing and the craft of choosing supplement rich food sources that sustain your body from the back to front. In this part, we will investigate the tasty universe of healthy sustenance, where taste and wellbeing entwine to make an orchestra of flavors that charms the faculties and stimulates the spirit.

1. The Supplement Rich Symphony

At the core of supporting your body lies the ensemble of supplement rich food sources that offer a plentiful cluster of nutrients, minerals, and cell reinforcements. Embrace the energetic shades of nature's abundance with an overflow of foods grown from the ground, each with a novel range of supplements supporting your prosperity. Appreciate the healthy integrity of entire grains, lean proteins, and sound fats, as they sustain your body with fundamental supplements, leaving you feeling fed and strengthened.

2. Hydration: The Solution of Life

Water, the solution of life, is the underpinning of sustaining your body. More than just quenching thirst, hydration is essential; It is essential for maintaining optimal body functions, including digestion, circulation, temperature control, and mental clarity. Embrace the propensity for tasting water over the course of the day, and supplement it with natural teas, implanted waters, and hydrating organic products to keep your body's stream of life streaming plentifully.

3. Embracing the Force of Superfoods

Superfoods, nature's wholesome forces to be reckoned with, are a stunning group of stars of food sources that offer a remarkable centralization of medical advantages. From supplement pressed berries to omega-3 rich chia seeds and cell reinforcement rich dull salad greens, these hotshots can lift your culinary manifestations higher than ever of sustenance and taste. Embrace the marvel of superfoods as you imbue your feasts with an additional portion of wellbeing improving properties.

4. The Art of Mindful Eating. The art of mindful eating, a transformative practice that enhances your dining experiences and fosters a deeper connection with the food you consume, lies beyond the nutritional value of food. Embrace the delight of enjoying each chomp, savoring the surfaces and flavors that dance on your taste buds, and connecting every one of your faculties to completely see the value in the culinary excursion you set out upon.

5. An Ensemble of Balance

In the amazing ensemble of feeding your body, balance is the director that coordinates your culinary wellbeing. Embrace the substance of balance as you enjoy periodic treats while focusing on supplementing thick food varieties. Recall that sustenance isn't about hardship yet about finding congruence among wellbeing and pleasure, relishing the different cluster of food sources that advance your life.

Conclusion
 Nourishing your body is a magnificent culinary adventure, a wellness journey that celebrates the art of nutritious nutrition and the pleasure of mindful eating. As you set out on this experience, let the lively varieties, tempting flavors, and feeding food be your manual for an existence of imperativeness and prosperity. Take advantage of the gift of culinary wellness because it is the key to a health symphony in which every bite is a

delicious masterpiece that nourishes your body and soul. Bon appétit!

3.1 Supplement Rich Food sources for Ideal Wellbeing: Relish the Abundance of Nature's Nourishment

In the charming domain of solid living, supplement rich food varieties stand as nature's bountiful gifts, offering a mother lode of nutrients, minerals, and fundamental mixtures that fuel our bodies with essentialness and strength. Like a thriving nursery, these food varieties paint a lively range of varieties, each tint addressing a one of a kind mix of wellbeing improving properties. We invite you to savor the bounty and embrace the art of nourishing your body for optimal health in this delectable journey through the world of nutrient-rich foods.

1. The Rainbow of Products of the soil

A clear rainbow of foods grown from the ground anticipates, each shade a demonstration of the range of supplements it gives. From the fiery oranges and delicious berries, overflowing with L-ascorbic acid and cell reinforcements, to the mixed greens and lavishly hued vegetables abounding with nutrients A, K, and minerals like iron and calcium. Take pleasure in the various flavors and textures of these healthy wonders because they help boost immunity, improve digestion, and produce radiant skin.

2. The Healthy Decency of Entire Grains

Entire grains, the good groundwork of sustenance, effortlessly our plates with an abundance of fiber, nutrients, and minerals. Whether it's nutty quinoa, supplement stuffed earthy colored rice, or good oats, these grains fuel our bodies with supported energy and supporting stomach related wellbeing. Whole grains have a significant impact on heart health and blood sugar stability, so take pleasure in their earthy flavors and reassuring textures.

3. The Protein Powerhouses
As the essential components of a healthy body, lean proteins take center stage. Whether it's the delicious delicacy of fish and poultry, the hearty integrity of vegetables, or the healthy protein-pressed seeds like chia and hemp, these forces to be reckoned with fuel our muscles, support cell fix, and keep up with solid skin, hair, and nails. Embrace the delicious variety of proteins as you relish the flavors that sustain your body with strength and versatility.

4. The Sound Fats that Nourish

In the nursery of sustenance, sound fats bloom like sensitive blossoms, offering fundamental unsaturated fats that help cerebrum wellbeing, diminish irritation, and keep up with flexible skin. These fats nourish your body's most important functions, from the luscious avocados and velvety richness of nuts to the golden drizzle of extra-virgin olive oil, adding depth and flavor to your meals.

5. The Enchantment of Flavors and Herbs

In the midst of the supplement rich abundance, flavors and spices add a bit of wizardry to our culinary manifestations. These treasures have powerful antioxidant and anti-inflammatory properties in addition to their delightful aromas and flavors. Embrace the fragrant orchestra of cinnamon, the fiery charm of turmeric, and the reviving substance of mint as they imbue your dishes with wellbeing upgrading benefits.

Conclusion

The universe of supplement rich food varieties is a meal of lively flavors and life-improving food. As you venture through this different scene, recollect that each chomp is a chance to support your body and embrace ideal wellbeing. Let each meal become a celebration of nourishment and well-being by savoring the colors, textures, and aromas that nature bestows upon us. Embrace the specialty of enjoying the abundance of supplement rich food sources, for in their tasty hug lies the way into an existence of imperativeness, strength, and enduring wellbeing. Bon appétit!

3.2 Hydration and Its Effect on Prosperity: Extinguishing the Body's Hunger for Vitality

In the orchestra of solid living, hydration remains as the reviving tune that fits our bodies, supporting each cell and framework with life-supporting water. Like a streaming waterway, hydration extinguishes the body's hunger for essentialness, affecting our physical, mental, and close to home prosperity in significant ways. This section examines the fundamentals of hydration and its significant impact on our overall health and vitality.

1. The Essential Job of Water

Water, the mixture of life, shapes the actual quintessence of hydration. Containing over a portion of our body weight, water assumes an imperative part in essentially every important physical process. It aids in digestion, transports nutrients and oxygen, regulates body temperature, and eliminates waste products. Accept the mental clarity that comes from drinking enough water because it keeps the brain sharp and focused.

2. Maintaining a Balance of Fluids. For optimal health, it is essential to keep the body's fluid levels in a delicate balance. Fatigue, headaches, impaired cognitive function, and kidney stress are all symptoms of dehydration. Be consistent in drinking water throughout the day, pay attention to your body's signals that it is

thirsty, and understand the significance of maintaining a healthy fluid balance.

3. Helping Actual Performance

For the individuals who lead a functioning way of life, appropriate hydration is the way to opening pinnacle actual execution. Remaining hydrated during exercise upgrades bloodstream to muscles, controls internal heat level, and forestalls squeezing and weakness. Maintaining adequate hydration throughout your workouts will give you the feeling of increased endurance and stamina.

4. Maintaining Digestive Health. Proper hydration is essential for maintaining regular bowel movements and digestive health. Water helps with the breakdown and ingestion of supplements, guaranteeing that your body can effectively use the sustenance from the food sources you polish off. Embrace the solace of a very much hydrated stomach related framework, as it advances legitimate supplement retention and decreases the probability of stoppage.

5. Beauty and radiant skin. Hydrated skin is radiant skin. Water reduces the appearance of fine lines and wrinkles by maintaining skin's elasticity and plumpness. Knowing that your skin is being fed from the inside out, take pleasure in the natural glow that results from maintaining adequate hydration.

6. Mental Lucidity and Close to home Well-being

Past the actual advantages, hydration significantly influences our psychological lucidity and close to home prosperity. Keeping hydrated aids in mood and cognitive function, preventing fogginess and improving focus. Embrace the feeling of mental readiness and profound equilibrium that goes with appropriate hydration.

Conclusion

Hydration is a strong power that rejuvenates our bodies, supporting our physical, mental, and close to home prosperity. Keep in mind the numerous advantages of drinking enough water as you adopt the habit of staying hydrated. Like a cool beverage on a warm summer day, hydration extinguishes the body's hunger for imperativeness, invigorating each part of your life. Relish the basic yet significant demonstration of drinking water, knowing that with each taste, you support your body, revive your psyche, and renew your soul. We salute the delightful journey of hydration and its numerous advantages!

3.3 Superfoods' potency: Releasing Nature's Nourishing Marvels

In the enrapturing embroidery of solid living, superfoods arise as nature's dietary wonders - a class of exceptional food varieties that rise above the normal, offering a mother lode of wellbeing upgrading benefits. Like enormous jewels in a tremendous universe, these superfoods gleam with a wealth of supplements, cell reinforcements, and phytochemicals, giving us an ensemble of prosperity. In this segment, we leave on a striking excursion to investigate the force of superfoods, opening the mysteries they hold for essentialness and ideal wellbeing.

1. A Bounty of Antioxidants
 A bounty of remarkable compounds that protect our bodies from oxidative stress and cellular damage are at the heart of superfoods. From the dazzling blueberries and lively pomegranates to the smooth dim chocolate and verdant spinach, these food sources are authentic gatekeepers of wellbeing, killing free revolutionaries and advancing cell revival.

2. Supporting Heart Health

Superfoods stand as impressive partners in the journey for heart wellbeing. In order to support cardiovascular function and maintain healthy cholesterol levels, the nutrient-dense berries and luscious avocados, which are full of heart-healthy monounsaturated fats, work together. Knowing that each superfood contributes its own special benefits to the orchestra of cardiovascular health, embrace the culinary art of feeding your heart.

3. Enhancing Cognitive Function and Promoting Clarity of Thought. The power of superfoods extends to brain

health. Among the culinary treasures that give our minds vitality are walnuts, which are high in omega-3 fatty acids, and turmeric, which helps the brain. Embrace the sustenance of your cerebrum as you appreciate the flavors that hone your smartness.

4. Building Solid Bones

In the ensemble of superfoods, calcium-rich kale and sesame seeds assume a main part in keeping up with bone wellbeing and forestalling osteoporosis. Embrace the strength that accompanies feeding your bones, knowing that these superfoods brace your skeletal design and backing in general outer muscle prosperity.

5. Adjusting Glucose Levels

For those looking to adjust glucose levels, the vegetable top dog chickpeas and the fiber-rich quinoa become the overwhelming focus in the realm of superfoods. Embrace the delight of stable energy levels and further developed insulin responsiveness, as these food sources assist with controlling glucose and add to a reasonable eating regimen.

6. The Marvel of Adaptogens. The magical class of superfoods known as adaptogens possess the capacity to adapt to the requirements of the body, assisting in stress reduction and restoring equilibrium. From the adaptogenic miracles of ashwagandha and heavenly basil to the quieting embrace of chamomile, these

superfoods support the body's pressure reaction, advancing strength and profound prosperity.

Conclusion

The force of superfoods is a disclosure, an orchestra of sustenance that raises our wellbeing and prosperity higher than ever. As you venture through the universe of supplement thick superfoods, recall that each culinary diamond carries its one of a kind gift to improve your essentialness. Embrace the flavors, varieties, and surfaces of these phenomenal food varieties, knowing that with each nibble, you are sustaining your body and soul. The universe of superfoods welcomes you to participate in this culinary experience, where taste and wellbeing join together, and the advantages of ideal sustenance embrace you in an orchestra of prosperity. Thus, let the banquet start, and may the force of superfoods enlighten your way to an existence of energetic well being and essentialness!

CONTENT 4

Planning for an Active Lifestyle:

Light the Flash of Imperativeness, Embrace the Delight of Movement

In the domain of solid carrying on with, dynamic way of life systems light the flash of imperativeness, coaxing us to embrace the delight of development and open the maximum capacity of our bodies. A long way past the limits of a repetitive exercise routine daily schedule, these procedures incorporate a dynamic and invigorating excursion, enabling us to implant every day with intentional movement and actual commitment. The keys to a life of vibrancy, strength, and lasting well-being are unveiled in this section, as we begin an invigorating look at active lifestyle strategies.

1. Discover the Pleasure of Movement. The discovery of pleasure in movement is at the heart of active lifestyle strategies. Dumping the thought of activity as a task, we embrace the freeing thought that development is a festival of our body's capacities. Participate in exercises that light your enthusiasm, whether it's moving, climbing, cycling, or playing a game you love. Relish the delight of moving your body, and let each step and each breath become a demonstration of the essentialness inside you.

2. Include Physical Activity on a Daily Basis
Adopting an active lifestyle necessitates more than just scheduled workouts. It's an invitation to get active on a regular basis. Engage in active play with family and friends, take the stairs rather than the elevator, walk or bike to nearby locations, stand up and stretch throughout the day. Embrace the endowment of development in each second, meshing active work into the texture of your life.

3. Embrace the Great Outdoors

Nature, a majestic canvas of wonder, exhorts us to use the great outdoors as a place to physically engage. Outdoor activities boost our spirits and refresh our minds, whether we're jogging along scenic trails, kayaking in tranquil waters, or hiking through lush forests. Allow nature's beauty to inspire your active endeavors and embrace its healing power.

4. Strength Preparing for Empowerment

In the ensemble of dynamic way of life procedures, strength preparing remains as the crescendo that engages our bodies with versatility and utilitarian strength. Lifting loads, rehearsing bodyweight works out, or taking part in obstruction preparing tones our muscles as well as improves bone thickness and supports joint wellbeing. Embrace the feeling of strengthening that accompanies fabricating major areas of strength for a proficient body.

5. Track down Help and Accountability

Setting out on a functioning way of life excursion can be improved by the help and responsibility of similar people. Find people who share your enthusiasm for movement by joining a fitness class, sports club, or online community. Embrace the kinship and support as you cheer each other on towards your wellness objectives.

6. Respect Your Body's Need for Rest and Recovery
When pursuing an active lifestyle, it is essential to respect your body's need for rest and recovery. Recognize that adequate rest and quality sleep are essential for muscle repair, energy replenishment, and overall well-being, and embrace the wisdom of self-care.

Conclusion

Dynamic way of life methodologies are the doorway to an existence of energy and essentialness, an agreeable dance among development and prosperity. As you embrace the delight of development, let each step and each activity become a declaration of your obligation to a better, more joyful you. You are invited to awaken the dormant spark within yourself, to infuse your life with purposeful activity, and to embrace the liberating sense of vitality that comes with each movement in the world of active lifestyle strategies. In this way, make the most of every opportunity, let the delight of development lead the way, and set out on an extraordinary excursion towards an existence of solidarity, bliss, and enduring prosperity. Let the symphony of an active lifestyle continue because the melody of a successful and fulfilled life lies in its exhilarating cadence.

4.1 Tomfoolery and Compelling Gym routine Schedules: Release Your Internal Wellness Enthusiast

In the enthralling domain of sound living, fun and compelling gym routine schedules arise as a definitive combination of wellness and bliss, welcoming us to release our internal wellness lovers and embrace the elation of development. The days of repetitive exercises are over; Our fitness journey is given new life by these routines, which give it energy, variety, and a sense of accomplishment. We begin an electrifying look at fun and effective workout routines in this section, revealing

the secrets to a fitness routine that revs us up and
makes us want more.

1. Dance Your Direction to Fitness

Step onto the dance floor and feel the musicality light
your spirit as you dance your direction to wellness.
Dance classes offer a wonderful combination of cardio
and self-expression, and they range from high-energy
Zumba classes to soulful hip-hop classes and graceful
ballet-inspired workouts. Embrace the freeing sensation
of moving your body to the music, and witness how
wellness turns into a dance of euphoria.

2. High-Intensity Interval Training, or HIIT for short, is a
powerful workout method that combines short bursts of
intense exercise with brief periods of rest. This
productive and compelling methodology lights calories,
helps digestion, and works on cardiovascular
perseverance. Embrace the test and fervor of stretching
your boundaries in spans, as you receive the benefits of
a fitter and more grounded you.

3. Experience of Outside Workouts

Nature's jungle gym coaxes us as we adventure into the
experience of outside exercises. Whether it's going
through picturesque scenes, paddleboarding on serene
waters, or rehearsing yoga in the recreation area, open
air exercises stimulate our spirits and associate us with
the excellence of nature. Embrace the excitement of

nature's hug, and let your wellness process become an elating outside caper.

4. Quieting Tranquility of Yoga

Yoga, an amicable orchestra of body, psyche, and breath, offers a peaceful desert spring amidst our bustling lives. Embrace the quieting tranquility of yoga as you course through asanas, developing strength, adaptability, and internal harmony. From delicate helpful practices to stimulating power yoga, the flexibility of yoga guarantees there's a style for everybody to embrace and appreciate.

5. Useful Preparation and Bodyweight Workouts

Bid goodbye to cumbersome hardware and embrace the force of practical preparation and bodyweight exercises. These schedules center around utilizing your body's regular developments to develop fortitude, strength, and adaptability. Embrace the comfort of exercises that should be possible anyplace, whenever, without the requirement for particular stuff. Your body turns into your definitive wellness instrument.

6. Interactive and Playful Fitness Games.

With interactive fitness games, why not make exercise a fun adventure? From computer generated reality wellness encounters to wellness based computer games, innovation welcomes us to consolidate amusement with work out. Embrace the delight of drawing in your brain and body in energetic difficulties, changing exercises into a thrilling and vivid experience.

Conclusion

Fun and powerful gym routine schedules are a passage to a wellness venture that exceeds all rational limitations. Let each workout be a celebration of your body's capabilities and a demonstration of your commitment to a healthier, happier you as you immerse yourself in the exciting workout world. Knowing that each step, every movement, and every moment of exhilaration brings you closer to your fitness goals, embrace the combination of fitness and joy. You are invited to unleash your inner fitness enthusiast, discover the thrill of pushing your limits, and experience the transformation that comes from embracing movement as an exhilarating adventure in the world of fun and effective workout routines. In this way, let the excursion start, and let the delight of wellness be your steadfast friend as you leave on an existence of essentialness, strength, and limitless energy for a better you.

4.2 Structure Solid Propensities for Day to day Development: Embrace the Excursion Towards a Functioning Lifestyle

In the domain of sound living, building solid propensities for day to day development is the groundbreaking pathway that guides us towards a functioning way of life loaded up with imperativeness and prosperity. Like the consistent progression of a waterway, these propensities bring us as the day progresses, imbuing it with intentional movement and empowering snapshots of actual commitment. In this segment, we set out on an engaging excursion to develop sound propensities that make development a vital piece of our regular routines, cultivating an amicable relationship with our bodies and a feeling of achievement.

1. Start with Small, Achievable Objectives
 As you begin the process of developing healthy routines for daily movement, recognize the value of taking baby steps. Start with reachable objectives that fit consistently into your ongoing daily practice. Whether you choose to walk for a few minutes during your lunch break, stretch for a few minutes in the morning, or take the stairs rather than the elevator, these small acts of movement build momentum and lay the groundwork for long-lasting habits.

2. Schedule Movement Breaks
 Just like you would for important appointments, incorporate movement breaks into your daily schedule. Put away committed time for active work, whether it's a speedy exercise, a dance meeting, or a yoga practice. Embrace the discipline of regarding these meetings with yourself, and witness how these purposeful breaks lift your energy and efficiency over the course of the day.

3. Track down Satisfaction in Dynamic Hobbies

Find dynamic side interests that light your energy and give pleasure to your life. In addition to adding movement to your day, participating in activities like gardening, biking, swimming, or sports also infuses it with contentment and happiness. Embrace the delight of seeking after side interests that sustain your spirit while keeping your body dynamic and lively.

4. Make Development a Social Experience

Embrace the force of social association as you fabricate solid propensities for day to day development. Join wellness classes, bunch exercises, or sports clubs to appreciate actual work with similar people. Participating in development with others encourages fellowship and responsibility, making the excursion towards a functioning way of life a common and elevating experience.

5. Focus on Dynamic Commuting

Rethink your everyday drive by consolidating dynamic transportation strategies. Walk or bicycle to work, go for public transportation and stroll to your objective, or park farther away from your objective to add additional moves toward your day. Embrace the potential chance to move your body while limiting your carbon impression and embracing a better and more economical way of life.

6. Observe Your Progress

Embrace the act of self-sympathy and praise your advancement en route. Building solid propensities for day to day development is an excursion of development, and each step in the right direction is a victory. Be kind to yourself when you fail, celebrate your accomplishments, and acknowledge your efforts. Believe that every day is a chance to start over and make choices that are good for your health.

Conclusion: A transformative journey of self-discovery and empowerment is developing healthy routines for daily movement. As you develop these propensities, recall that each step, regardless of how little, carries you more like a functioning way of life loaded up with essentialness and satisfaction. Embrace the excursion, for it is a festival of your obligation to supporting your body and embracing the endowment of development. With every day, you'll observe the change of solid propensities into an agreeable orchestra of prosperity, injecting your existence with energy, reason, and a more profound association with your body. Therefore, take that first step right now and let the road to a life that is both active and fulfilling unfold before you.

4.3 Getting Active Outside: Find the Excitement of Nature's Playground

In the charming domain of sound living, embracing outside exercises makes the way for a universe of experience and association with nature's grand jungle gym. Past the limits of indoor spaces, nature calls, welcoming us to delight in the magnificence of open scenes, take in the fresh air, and drench ourselves in the miracles of the regular world. In this segment, we set out on an elating excursion to find the excitement of open air exercises, lighting our spirits and supporting our bodies with the imperativeness of nature.

1. Hiking Scenic Trails

Enter the embrace of nature and embark on the enchantment of hiking scenic trails. Whether it's twisting ways through rich woodlands, stunning mountain trails, or waterfront strolls with clearing sea sees, climbing restores the spirit and fortifies the body. Embrace the delight of investigating new landscapes, relishing the excellence of the wild, and seeing the marvels of nature unfurl before your eyes.

2. Cycling on Nature's Pathways

Enjoy the freedom and rhythm of cycling along nature's paths as you pedal through tranquil landscapes. Whether on rough mountain trekking trails or smooth ways by the stream, cycling offers a tomfoolery and thrilling method for investigating nature while receiving the rewards of a full-body exercise. Embrace the breeze in your hair and the adventure of the excursion as you rediscover the delights of cycling.

3. Kayaking in Peaceful Waters
 As you embrace the adventure of kayaking in peaceful waters, step into a world of peace and tranquility. As you glide through tranquil lakes, gentle rivers, or coastal inlets, let the paddle's rhythmic motion bring you into harmony with nature's calming beat. Embrace the agreement of water and sky as you explore through nature's fluid pathways.

4. Setting up camp Under the Twilight Sky

Embrace the appeal of setting up camp as you adventure into nature and camp under the twilight sky. Setting up camp offers a getaway from the rushing about of day to day existence, permitting you to associate with nature's quiet hug. Embrace the delight of social occasions around an open air fire, sharing stories under the stars, and arousing the delicate beams of the sun as it ascends into the great beyond.

5. Yoga and meditation outdoors

 Bring your practice into the embrace of nature and enjoy the serenity of yoga and meditation outdoors. Yoga and meditation can be practiced outside, on a beach, in a park, or at the top of a hill with a view, allowing you to find stillness in the midst of nature's beauty. Embrace the feeling of establishing and restoration as you adjust your brain, body, and soul together as one with the normal world.

6. Embracing Nature's Elements

As you embrace open air exercises, make sure to regard and respect nature's components. Be mindful of environmental conservation, keep hydrated, and dress appropriately for the weather. Embrace the feeling of interconnectedness with the normal world, realizing that each step you make a move to support your prosperity and encourage a profound appreciation for the magnificence of nature.

Conclusion

Participating in activities in the great outdoors is a transformative journey of discovery and connection, a celebration of nature's grandeur, and a reconnection with our inherent love of the great outdoors. As you venture into the playground of nature, let each step be an invitation to rediscover the pleasures of outdoor adventure and an awakening of your senses. The universe of open air exercises anticipates, enticing you to investigate, restore, and sustain your body, psyche, and soul in the midst of the magnificence of the normal world. Therefore, let the excitement of outdoor activities direct you toward a life filled with vitality, wonder, and a profound appreciation for nature's gifts. On this transformative journey toward a life enriched by the wonders of nature, let the adventure begin, and may the great outdoors become your faithful companion.

CONTENT 5

Self-care and mental health: Sustaining the Asylum Within

In the hallowed safe-haven of sound living, psychological well-being and taking care of oneself entwine as the fundamental strings that weave the embroidered artwork of our prosperity. Past the actual domain, our psyches and feelings structure the foundation of an amicable presence. In this part, we leave on a spirit blending excursion to investigate the significant meaning of psychological wellness and taking care of oneself, finding the force of sustaining the safe-haven inside.

1. The Vitality of Mental Health

As the orchestrator of our emotional well-being, mental health takes center stage in the symphony of self-care. Taking care of our mental health is just as important as taking care of our physical health. Embrace the comprehension that psychological well-being incorporates a range of feelings and encounters, and that looking for help and direction when required is a brave demonstration of self-sympathy.

2. Self-care is an art that gently cradles our souls and encourages us to prioritize our well-being in the midst of life's demands. Whether it's taking a soothing bath, spending time in nature, writing in a journal, or engaging in a favorite pastime, self-care rituals are beautiful. Allow self-care to serve as a haven of tranquility and a reminder of your inherent worth.

3. The Recuperating Force of Mindfulness

In the quick moving dance of life, care arises as an extraordinary practice that grounds us right now. Embrace the endowment of care, permitting you to notice your considerations and sentiments without judgment. Develop care through contemplation, profound breathing, or careful development, and witness how this training upgrades your close to home versatility and encourages a profound feeling of internal harmony.

4. Honoring and Connecting with Our Emotions
 Embodiment of mental health and self-care necessitates honoring and connecting with our emotions. Permit yourself to experience and communicate a full scope of feelings, perceiving that they are regular and part of the human experience. Embrace the act of close to home mindfulness,

understanding that recognizing and handling feelings is a strong type of self-strengthening.

5. Developing Sound Relationships

The associations we produce with others assume a crucial part in our psychological prosperity. Embrace the act of developing solid connections, encircling yourself with strong and sustaining people who elevate and motivate you. Openly communicate with one another and make an effort to forge meaningful connections that will benefit your mental health.

6. Looking for Proficient Support

In the excursion towards mental prosperity, looking for proficient help can be groundbreaking. Reaching out to professionals in the field of mental health, whether through therapy, counseling, or support groups, provides helpful insights and strategies for overcoming obstacles in life. Recognize that taking the courageous step of seeking assistance when you need it is a strength that you should embrace.

Conclusion

Emotional well-being and taking care of oneself structure the groundwork of a decent and satisfying life, a safe-haven of prosperity where our brains and spirits track down comfort and flexibility. As you embrace the meaning of psychological wellness and taking care of oneself, let every second turn into a chance to sustain the safe-haven inside. Embrace the act of self-empathy, recognizing that you are meriting adoration and care. Allow care to be your aide, securing you in the present and permitting you to relish the magnificence of each passing second. The universe of emotional wellness and taking care of oneself welcomes you to set out on a spirit mixing venture, to embrace weakness as strength, and to find the groundbreaking force of sustaining the safe-haven inside. Thus, let taking care of oneself be your compass, and may the excursion towards mental prosperity lead you to an existence of satisfaction, happiness, and significant association with yourself as well as other people.

5.1 Making Self-Care a Priority in Your Schedule:

Embrace the Art of Nurturing Yourself** Prioritizing self-care emerges as the soul-stirring melody that harmonizes our mind, body, and spirit in the symphony of a fulfilling life. Like a delicate breeze that strokes our spirits, taking care of oneself sustains and restores us, permitting us to flourish in the midst of life's requests. In this part, we leave on an enabling excursion to investigate the specialty of focusing on taking care of oneself in your daily schedule, disclosing the extraordinary force of embracing snapshots of comfort and self-empathy.

1. Cutting Out Consecrated Time

In the midst of the clamoring beat of day to day existence, cut out hallowed time for taking care of oneself like a show-stopper etched from time's hug. As you would with any important commitment, schedule time for self-care as a non-negotiable appointment with yourself. Whether it's a couple of moments of contemplation in the first part of the day, a stroll in nature during lunch, or a night devoted to your number one leisure activity, let this time be a desert spring of comfort and restoration.

2. Embracing the Force of Saying "No"

Chasing, taking care of oneself, embracing the freeing craft of saying "no" to responsibilities that exhaust your energy and prosperity. Focus on your necessities and limits, understanding that taking care of oneself is a gift you present to yourself. By clearing out your schedule, you free up time for self-care and make sure you have the energy to focus on what really matters.

3. Finding Self-Compassion

Embrace the delicate hug of self-empathy as you venture through the scene of taking care of oneself. Indulge yourself with a similar thoughtfulness and understanding you would offer a dear companion. Discharge the heaviness of self-judgment, and on second thought, embrace the excellence of tolerating yourself as you are. Here of self esteem, you'll track down the opportunity to focus on your prosperity without culpability or faltering.

4. Making an Individual Taking care of oneself Ritual

Create an individual taking care of oneself custom that addresses your spirit and sustains your being. Embrace the lavishness of choices, from cozying up with a book and a warm cup of tea to spoiling yourself with a mitigating shower or participating in careful development. This ritual becomes your haven, a place to refuel your spirit and embrace the essence of self-care.

5. Connecting with Nature

 Nature, a limitless source of healing and inspiration, encourages us to prioritize self-care in its embrace. Embrace the quietness of investing energy outside, submerging yourself in the marvels of the normal world. Whether it's a comfortable walk around a recreation area, a climb in the mountains, or basically sitting under a tree, nature's excellence turns into the material whereupon you paint snapshots of serenity and reestablishment.

6. Rehearsing Gratitude

In the specialty of focusing on taking care of oneself, appreciation arises as a groundbreaking power. Embrace the act of appreciation, communicating appreciation for the snapshots of taking care of oneself and the gifts in your day to day existence. Create a gratitude journal in which you record the little pleasures and moments of comfort that you incorporate into your daily routine. This training enhances the force of taking care of oneself, helping you to remember the overflow that encompasses you.

Conclusion

Focusing on taking care of oneself in your routine is an ensemble of sustaining yourself, an engaging dance of self-sympathy, and a tribute to the magnificence of renewing your soul. Let each moment become a celebration of your inherent worthiness as you embrace the art of self-care. Accept the practice of putting yourself first, knowing that by taking care of yourself, you become better prepared to face life's challenges and appreciate its pleasures. The universe of taking care of oneself welcomes you to step into the safe-haven of your spirit, to make a day to day existence that praises your requirements and embraces snapshots of comfort. Therefore, allow the tune of self-care to lead you toward a life filled with vitality, equilibrium, and a profound connection to yourself. Embrace the excursion, for inside the specialty of taking care of oneself lies the way into an existence of satisfaction, euphoria, and unlimited prosperity.

5.2 Procedures for Stress Decrease: Opening the Way to Serenity

In the quick moving orchestra of present day life, procedures for stress decrease arise as the alleviating rhythm that reestablishes congruence to our psyches and bodies. These methods give us a break from the chaos and give us the ability to face life's challenges with grace and resilience, like a gentle breeze that calms the turbulent waves. In this section, we begin a life-altering journey to learn about the art of stress reduction and discover the power of embracing moments of inner peace and serenity.

1. Mindful Breathing

In the art of stress management, mindful breathing is the fundamental practice that brings us into the now. Take some time to focus solely on your breath and enjoy the simplicity of this method. Feel the ascent and fall of your chest, the vibe of the air going through your noses. Relax and connect with your inner peace as you immerse yourself in the rhythm of your breath.

2. Reflection and Mindfulness

Embrace the significant act of reflection and care as you adventure into the domain of stress. These practices invite you to observe your thoughts and feelings with gentle acceptance, whether through guided meditations, body scans, or mindfulness exercises. In the asylum of contemplation, you find a desert garden of quiet in the midst of life's disturbance.

3. Getting Active

Getting active is a great way to reduce stress because it helps the body release endorphins, which are natural stress-busters. Embrace the delight of development, whether it's a comfortable walk, a heart-siphoning exercise, or a dance meeting. Physical activity not only reduces stress but also improves your physical health, giving you a sense of vitality and equilibrium.

4. Supporting Nature's Embrace

Nature, a plentiful wellspring of comfort and reestablishment, coaxes us to look for shelter in its hug. Embrace the mending force of nature as you invest energy outside, whether it's getting out in the forest, reflecting by the ocean side, or just lounging in the daylight. In nature's safe-haven, you find a safe-haven that renews your soul and reestablishes your feeling of association with your general surroundings.

5. Cultivating Gratitude

Gratitude, a transformative force, injects a sense of abundance and contentment into the art of stress reduction. Whether you do it in the form of daily reflections or journaling, embrace the practice of gratitude and acknowledge the joys and blessings in your life. As you develop appreciation, you shift your concentration from stressors to the gifts that encompass you.

6. Taking part in Imaginative Expression

Imaginative articulation, a soothing source for feelings, encourages pressure decrease through the innovative stream. Participating in creative endeavors, such as painting, writing, music, or crafting, is a joy to behold. You transcend stress and find solace in the beauty of self-expression as you immerse yourself in the act of creation.

Conclusion

Techniques for reducing stress are a calming symphony and an empowering dance that help us overcome obstacles in life with grace and resilience. As you embrace these methods, let every second be a valuable chance to deliver pressure, track down comfort in the present, and cultivate a more profound association with yourself. Stress decrease turns into an extraordinary excursion, a way that drives you to embrace internal harmony in the midst of the bedlam of life. Thus, let the songs of careful breathing, reflection, actual work, and innovative articulation guide you towards an existence of peacefulness and strengthening. Embrace the specialty of stress decrease, and may it become a dependable friend on your excursion to an existence of unlimited prosperity and significant serenity.

5.3 Improving Resilience to Emotional Stress:

Enhancing emotional resilience emerges as the awe-inspiring brushstroke that imbues us with inner strength and fortitude on the canvas of life's intricate tapestry. Like a glorious oak facing hardships, close to home flexibility engages us to explore life's difficulties with boldness and beauty. In this segment, we set out on an extraordinary excursion to investigate the specialty of improving close to home flexibility, divulging the significant force of embracing our feelings and developing versatility notwithstanding misfortune.

1. Embracing the Range of Emotions

At the core of close to home strength lies the significant craft of embracing the range of feelings. Permit yourself to encounter a full scope of sentiments, recognizing that they are a characteristic piece of being human. Embrace the act of profound mindfulness, perceiving your feelings without judgment. By regarding your sentiments, you leave on an excursion of self-empathy and realness.

2. Building a Strong Network

The strength of close to home versatility is enhanced by the help of a supporting organization. Encircle yourself with strong and understanding people who offer a place of refuge for you to communicate your sentiments and look for direction when required. Embrace the force of weakness, realizing that resting on others is a valiant demonstration that encourages association and profound strength.

3. Developing Self-Compassion

In the craft of upgrading profound flexibility, self-empathy turns into the delicate salve that mends and sustains our spirits. Indulge yourself with generosity and understanding, offering a similar empathy you would stretch out to a dear companion. Accept that imperfections are a beautiful aspect of the human experience and that it is acceptable to feel vulnerable.

4. Adopting a Growth Mindset

 Recognize that difficulties present opportunities for development and learning and embrace the empowering belief in a growth mindset. Develop a positive outlook on adversity and view setbacks as stepping stones rather than obstacles. You can turn challenges into opportunities for resilience and personal development by adopting a growth mindset.

5. Taking part in Pressure Decreasing Practices

Stress-decreasing practices, similar to contemplation, care, and active work, encourage close to home versatility by quieting the brain and calming the soul. Embrace the force of these works on, permitting them to become mainstays of solidarity in the midst of life's tempests. As you participate in pressure lessening exercises, you support your close to home prosperity and make a groundwork of inward strength.

6. Embracing Adaptability and Adaptability

In the orchestra of profound strength, adaptability and versatility structure the amicable tune that empowers us to explore life's consistently evolving scene. Embrace the comprehension that life is erratic, and difficulties will emerge. Embracing adaptability and flexibility permits you to stream with life's ebbs and flows, changing affliction into a chance for development and advancement.

Conclusion

Improving close to home flexibility is an enabling excursion of internal strength, a dance of genuineness, and a demonstration of the magnificence of weakness. As you embrace profound flexibility, let every second be a potential chance to develop self-sympathy, fabricate a strong organization, and take part in rehearsals that support your prosperity. A symphony of inner strength, emotional resilience develops into a transformative art that enables you to face life's challenges with grace and fortitude. In this way, let the tunes of weakness, self-empathy, and development guide you towards an existence of profound versatility, realizing that inside the specialty of flexibility lies the way into an existence of legitimacy, fortitude, and limitless inward strength.

CONTENT 6

Quality Rest and Rest: The Reviving Ensemble of Rejuvenation

In the terrific ensemble of sound living, quality rest and rest arise as the amicable notes that weave the texture of our prosperity. Like a supportive bedtime song, these components embrace us with quietness, feeding our bodies and psyches, and setting us up to embrace each new day with life and essentialness. In this section, we embark on a transformative journey to discover the profound power of surrendering to the calming embrace of rejuvenation and the art of quality sleep and rest.

1. Embracing the Mixture of Sleep

Inside the domain of value rest and rest lies the mixture of life - rest. Embrace the comprehension that rest isn't an extravagance however a fundamental part of our physical and psychological well-being. Recognizing that your body heals, restores, and prepares for the day ahead while you sleep, give your sleep the same importance as you would any other important aspect of your life, prioritize it.

2. Making a Quiet Rest Environment

Change your rest climate into a safe-haven of quietness. Embrace the mitigating force of an agreeable sleeping pad and cushions, power outage shades to shut out light, and a quieting variety plot that cultivates unwinding. Eliminate electronic gadgets that transmit invigorating blue light and make a space helpful for serene sleep.

3. Embracing Predictable Rest Schedule

In the craft of value rest, consistency is the guide that guarantees an amicable musicality. Embrace the act of an ordinary rest plan, heading to sleep and awakening simultaneously every day, even at the end of the week. You can improve the quality of your sleep and your overall well-being by embracing consistency and synchronizing your internal body clock.

4. Embracing the enchantment of bedtime rituals, which signal to your mind and body that it's time to unwind, Before going to bed, engage in calming activities like reading, doing gentle yoga, or meditating. Preparing yourself for a restful night's sleep, allows your mind to transition from the busyness of the day to a state of tranquility.

5. Restricting Energizers and Screens

Chasing quality rest, embrace the act of restricting energizers and screen time near sleep time. Keep away from caffeine and weighty dinners before rest, as they can upset your capacity to nod off. Limit screen openness to essentially an hour prior to bed, as the blue light produced by screens can disrupt your body's normal rest wake cycle.

6. Respecting Your Rest Needs

Embrace the craft of paying attention to your body's rest needs. Know that rest includes taking breaks and allowing yourself to recharge throughout the day in addition to sleeping. Embrace the act of soothing exercises, like investing energy in nature, rehearsing care, or taking part in leisure activities that give you pleasure.

Conclusion

Quality rest and rest are the songs that revive our bodies and support our psyches, an agreeable orchestra of prosperity. As you embrace the craft of value rest and rest, let every night be a potential chance to give up to the hug of revival and every day a festival of reestablished imperativeness. Embrace the force of steady rest propensities, a quiet rest climate, and sleep time customs that set you up for tranquil sleep. Inside the craft of value rest and rest lies the way into an existence of imperativeness, clearness, and limitless prosperity. In this way, let the orchestra of revival guide you towards an existence of peaceful evenings and rejuvenated days, realizing that inside the hug of value rest and rest lies the significant ability to carry on with life to its fullest potential.

6.1 Grasping the Significance of Rest: Unwinding the Secrets of a Helpful Journey

In the enrapturing domain of sound living, rest becomes the dominant focal point as the captivating journey that revives our bodies, upgrades our mental capacities, and sustains our close to home prosperity. Our minds and bodies embark on a profound exploration of rejuvenation during a restorative journey that goes beyond a simple period of rest. The transformative power of this nightly ritual is illuminated as we delve into the depths of understanding the significance of sleep in this section.

1. The Power of Restorative Sleep

Sleep, like a magical potion, holds the key to renewal and restoration. During rest, our bodies go through fundamental cycles of fix, development, and safe framework reinforcing. In order to speed up growth and healing, tissues are regenerated, muscles are fixed, and hormones are released. Embrace the comprehension that quality rest is the underpinning of generally prosperity, permitting you to get up every early daytime feeling invigorated and prepared to embrace the day.

2. Upgrading Mental Function

Past actual rebuilding, rest upgrades our mental capability, honing our smartness and supporting our imagination. During rest, our minds combine recollections and interaction data assembled during the day, prompting further developed learning and critical thinking skills. Accept the confidence-boosting knowledge that getting enough quality sleep is not only good for our bodies but also good for our minds, helping us develop our cognitive abilities and maintain optimal brain health.

3. Adjusting Close to home Well-being

In the domain of rest's significance lies its significant effect on close to home prosperity. Sufficient rest upholds profound guidelines, assisting us with overseeing pressure and keeping an uplifting perspective on life. On the other hand, not getting enough sleep can cause mood swings, irritability, and an increased risk of anxiety and depression. Accept that getting enough quality sleep helps you maintain emotional equilibrium, allowing you to overcome obstacles in life with resiliency and clarity.

4. Supporting Actual Health

The meaning of rest reaches out to our actual wellbeing, assuming a vital part in keeping a solid safe framework and supporting cardiovascular wellbeing. Obesity, diabetes, and heart disease are just a few of the health issues that are linked to chronic sleep deprivation. Take comfort in the knowledge that getting a good night's sleep is an important investment in your long-term health and vitality.

5. Working with Chemical Regulation

Inside the craft of rest lies the multifaceted dance of chemical guidelines. The release of various hormones that regulate appetite, metabolism, and stress responses is directly influenced by sleep. Accept the fact that getting enough sleep helps maintain a healthy hormone balance, which aids in weight management and overall metabolic health.

6. Unwinding the Secrets of Dreams

Rest holds the captivating appeal of dreams, where our psyche minds leave on innovative excursions. Dreaming is accepted to assume a part in profound handling, memory combination, and imagination. Embrace the interest of dreams, remembering them as a fundamental piece of the perplexing embroidered artwork of rest's significance.

Conclusion

Understanding the significance of rest reveals the extraordinary force of this helpful excursion that we leave on every evening. Let each night be a treasured opportunity to surrender to the embrace of rejuvenation and each morning be a celebration of renewed vitality as you embrace the significance of sleep. Embrace the comprehension that rest isn't only a time of rest however a significant investigation of physical, mental, and close to home revival. The key to a life filled with vitality, clarity, and limitless well-being is good sleep. In this way, let the secrets of rest guide you towards an existence of tranquil evenings and renewed days, realizing that inside the craft of rest lies the significant ability to carry on with life to its fullest potential.

6.2 Further developing Rest Cleanliness for Better Rest: Creating a Quiet Sleep Sanctuary

In the charming quest for solid living, further developing rest cleanliness arises as the captivating craftsmanship that changes our evenings into soothing safe-havens of revival. Sleep hygiene wraps us in the embrace of optimal sleep practices, lulling us to sleep like a soft lullaby, enabling us to feel refreshed and alive each morning. In this segment, we set out on an engaging excursion to investigate the specialty of further developing rest cleanliness, divulging the groundbreaking force of creating a tranquil sleep safe-haven for better rest.

1. Embrace a Consistent Sleep Schedule

The rhythmic melody of a consistent sleep schedule is at the heart of improving sleep hygiene. Embrace the engaging act of heading to sleep and awakening simultaneously every day, even at the end of the week. By regarding your body's normal rest wake cycle, you synchronize your inner clock, advancing better rest quality and by and large prosperity.

2. Make a Rest Instigating Environment

Change your rest climate into a safe house of quietness. Make use of white noise machines and blackout curtains when necessary to practice the art of minimizing light and noise pollution. Keep your rest space cool, as a marginally lower temperature is helpful for better rest. Create a rest-inciting climate that welcomes tranquil sleep and unwinding.

3. Limit stimulating activities before bed

If you want to get a better night's sleep, try doing calming activities before bed. Close to bedtime, avoid stimulating activities like watching violent movies or having discussions that are emotionally charged. To prepare your mind and body for restful sleep, instead, indulge in calming rituals like reading a book, gentle yoga, or taking a warm bath.

4. Limit Screen Time Before Bed

Inside the domain of rest cleanliness lies the agreeable act of restricting screen time before bed. The blue light that comes from electronic devices can make it hard for our bodies to make melatonin, the hormone that helps us sleep, on their own. Embrace the engaging demonstration of disengaging from screens essentially an hour prior to sleep time, permitting your psyche to loosen up and plan for sleep.

5. Sustain with Rest Steady Foods

In the orchestra of further developing rest cleanliness, sustaining your body with rest strong food varieties assumes a crucial part. Include foods that are high in nutrients that aid in sleep, like magnesium and tryptophan, in your evening meals. Food sources like bananas, almonds, and warm milk have relieving properties that improve unwinding and support better rest.

6. Embrace Pressure Decrease Techniques

Inside the craft of further developing rest cleanliness lies the engaging act of pressure decrease. To calm your mind and let go of tension, try stress-reduction methods like deep breathing, progressive muscle relaxation, or meditation. You can create a peaceful sleeping space by letting go of stress before bed.

Conclusion

Further developing rest cleanliness is an extraordinary excursion of creating a tranquil sleep safe-haven, a dance of steady rest plans, mitigating conditions, and quieting ceremonies. As you embrace the craft of rest cleanliness, let every night be a treasured open door to give up to the hug of revival and every morning a festival of reestablished essentialness. Embrace the comprehension that quality rest isn't just a time of rest yet a significant investigation of physical, mental, and close to home recharging. Inside the hug of further developed rest cleanliness lies the way into an existence of essentialness, clearness, and limitless prosperity. Therefore, with the knowledge that the profound power to live life to the fullest lies within the tranquil embrace of the art of sleep hygiene, allow it to guide you toward a life of restful nights and revitalized days.

6.3 Unwinding Procedures for More profound Rest: Unveiling the Doorway to Serenity

In the mesmerizing world of healthy living, relaxation techniques become the enchantment that leads to a world of peaceful sleep and more restful sleep. Like a delicate breeze that clears away the day's concerns, these procedures support us in quietness, permitting us to float into a significant condition of rest and revival. In this section, we embark on an engaging journey to discover the transformative power of surrendering to the embrace of serenity and the art of relaxation techniques for deeper sleep.

1. Moderate Muscle Relaxation

Inside the domain of unwinding strategies lies the engaging act of moderate muscle unwinding. Embrace this delicate procedure as you gradually tense and afterward discharge each muscle bunch in your body, beginning from your toes and moving gradually up to your head. By relinquishing actual pressure, you signal your body to embrace unwinding, making ready for more profound rest.

2. Guided Imagery and Visualization

Take a tranquil mental journey by embracing the captivating art of guided imagery and visualization. Connect with your faculties by envisioning peaceful scenes, for example, a quieting ocean side or a rich woods. Allow your mind to drift off into a peaceful slumber by taking in the sights, sounds, and sensations of this mental haven.

3. Breathing Procedures for Calmness

Chasing after more profound rest, the mood of your breath turns into the captivating guide of peacefulness. Embrace quieting breathing procedures, for example, diaphragmatic breathing or the 4-7-8 method, to dial back your pulse and enact the body's unwinding reaction. You open the door to sound sleep by synchronizing your breath with peace.

4. Care Meditation

Inside the craft of unwinding strategies lies the extraordinary act of care reflection. Embrace the current second, noticing your contemplations and sentiments without judgment. Before going to bed, practice mindfulness meditation to let go of the stresses of the day and focus on the present moment. By calming your brain, you make the space for more profound and more helpful rest.

5. Fragrance based treatment for Relaxation

In the dazzling domain of unwinding methods, the aromas of natural oils become the charming embodiment of serenity. Embrace fragrance based treatment as you mix your rest climate with quieting aromas like lavender, chamomile, or . You'll drift off to a more peaceful sleep as a result of the calming scents' ability to induce relaxation.

6. Delicate Music and White Noise

Inside the ensemble of unwinding methods lies the delicate tune of delicate music and background noise. Take advantage of the calming effects of soul-resonant music or natural sounds. Permit the delicate sounds to make a mood of tranquility, veiling any troublesome

commotions and directing you into a more profound
condition of rest.

Conclusion

 Relaxation techniques become the stars that guide us
to a world of profound rejuvenation and deeper sleep.
As you embrace these methods, let every night become
a valued open door to give up to the hug of quietness
and every morning a festival of reestablished
imperativeness. Embrace the comprehension that
unwinding strategies are not simply instruments for rest,
however extraordinary practices that support your
prosperity on various levels. Inside the specialty of
unwinding methods lies the way into an existence of
tranquil evenings and rejuvenated days, realizing that
inside the hug of serenity lies the significant ability to
carry on with life to its fullest potential. In this way, let the
charming universe of unwinding procedures guide you
towards an existence of serenity, lucidity, and limitless
prosperity.

CONTENT 7

Fitting a work-life balance: Supporting Amiability in the Orchestra of Living

In the orchestra of life's mind boggling tunes, adjusting work and life arises as the spirit mixing mood that blends our expert interests and individual prosperity. Like a director coordinating a work of art, finding balance between these two domains permits us to lead satisfying and amicable lives. We explore the art of balancing work and life on an empowering journey in this comprehensive guide, revealing the transformative power of cultivating harmony in the symphony of living.

1. Define Your Priorities

The empowering act of defining your priorities is at the heart of finding a balance between work and life. Think about the main thing to you - your own qualities, connections, and expert aspirations. Embrace the comprehension that you can't do everything, and going with purposeful decisions about how you designate your significant investment is fundamental for accomplishing balance.

2. Set Boundaries

The harmonious practice of setting boundaries falls under the category of achieving a work-life balance. Make sure that your personal and professional lives do not overlap by drawing clear lines between them. Honor your need for rest and rejuvenation and embrace the art of saying "no" to commitments that do not align with your priorities.

3. Make an Adaptable Work Environment

Embrace the force of adaptability in your workplace, if conceivable. If you want to better manage your personal commitments, you should negotiate flexible work hours or think about remote work options. You can adjust your work schedule to meet the demands of your life in a flexible work environment, resulting in a sense of balance between the two worlds.

4. Practice Time Management

The transformative skill of time management lies within the art of balancing work and life. Embrace successful time usage methods, for example, making day to day daily agendas, focusing on errands, and setting time limits for exercises. By dealing with your time productively, you advance efficiency and make space for recreation and special goals.

5. Embrace Care and Self-Care

Chasing, adjusting work and life, care and taking care of oneself become the directing stars that support your prosperity. Embrace the act of care to remain present in every second, decreasing pressure and expanding center. Focus on taking care of oneself's customs, like activity, reflection, or investing energy in nature, to re-energize and revive your psyche and body.

6. Cultivate Steady Relationships

Inside the orchestra of adjusting work and life lies the enabling trap of strong connections. Develop associations with companions, family, and partners who get it and regard your requirement for balance. Create a supportive network that supports your well-being by embracing open communication about your priorities and commitments with loved ones.

7. Figure out how to Delegate and Look for Help

Inside the specialty of adjusting work and life lies the insight of appointment and looking for help. Embrace the comprehension that you don't need to convey the heaviness of all obligations alone. At work, delegate responsibilities and turn to friends and family for help when you need it. You will avoid burnout and achieve balance when you accept assistance.

8. Practice Gratitude

Inside the domain of adjusting work and life lies the extraordinary act of appreciation. Embrace the specialty of offering thanks for the valuable open doors and endowments in your day to day existence, both actually and expertly. To cultivate a sense of contentment and fulfillment, keep a gratitude journal and reflect on the positive aspects of your work and personal experiences.

Conclusion

Adjusting work and life is a spirit mixing excursion of supporting congruity in the ensemble of living. As you embrace this craftsmanship, let every second turn into a chance to characterize your needs, put down stopping points, and develop an adaptable workplace. Embrace using time productively and care to upgrade efficiency while sustaining taking care of oneself and cultivating steady connections. The secret to a life filled with happiness, limitless well-being, and fulfillment is the art of balancing work and life. In this way, let the core values of equilibrium lead you towards an amicable presence, realizing that inside the hug of equilibrium lies the significant ability to carry on with life to its fullest potential.

7.1 Time Usage Tips for a Solid Way of life: Holding onto the Rules of Time and Well-Being

In the charming quest for a solid way of life, using time productively arises as the engaging guide that permits us to hold onto control of our days and sustain our prosperity. Mastering time management arranges our commitments and priorities, paving the way for a life of balance, vitality, and fulfillment like a skilled conductor. In this segment, we set out on a connection with excursion to investigate time usage tips for a sound way of life, divulging the extraordinary force of fitting time and prosperity.

1. Focus on Self-Care

At the core of using time productively for a solid way of life lies the enabling demonstration of focusing on taking care of oneself. Set aside a few minutes for exercises that sustain your brain, body, and soul, whether it's activity, reflection, side interests, or investing energy in nature. You lay the groundwork for your overall health and vitality by making self-care an unavoidable part of your daily routine.

2. Plan and Coordinate Your Day

Inside the domain of time usage tips, arranging and coordinating your day become the directing stars that upgrade efficiency and concentration. Embrace the act of making a day to day plan for the day, framing your undertakings and objectives. You will be able to complete essential tasks more quickly if you set priorities and break them down into smaller, more manageable tasks.

3. Embrace Time Blocking

Chasing using time effectively for a sound way of life, time obstructing turns into the enabling procedure that assigns explicit time allotments for various exercises. Set aside time for work, exercise, eating, taking a break, and personal pursuits. To maximize your energy and focus throughout the day and minimize distractions, embrace the structure of time blocking.

4. Stay away from Overcommitment

Inside the craft of time usage lies the extraordinary insight of keeping away from overcommitment. Be deliberate with your responsibilities, grasping your cutoff points and the benefit of leaving space for recreation and unwinding. Saying "no" to unnecessary commitments can have a positive impact on your well-being and your schedule.

5. Streamline and Delegate

In the fascinating field of time management, you can focus on what really matters by streamlining and delegating tasks. Recognize tedious or tedious errands that can be smoothed out or mechanized. Utilize the skill of delegation and enlist the assistance of coworkers or family members for tasks that can be shared. By smoothing out and designating, you make additional opportunities for exercises that add to a sound way of life.

6. Limit Screen Time and Distractions

The harmonious practice of limiting screen time and distractions is part of the symphony of time management advice. Put down stopping points for virtual entertainment and other advanced stages to forestall time wastage. Focus on your work or personal time in a distraction-free environment to increase productivity and mindfulness.

7. Plan Standard Breaks

Chasing using time productively for a solid way of life, planning standard breaks turns into the renewing interval that supports your prosperity. Embrace brief breaks over the course of the day to extend, inhale, or basically unwind. Give your body and mind a break, which will help you focus and be more productive overall.

8. Reflect and Adjust

The transformative power of reflection and adjustment is embedded in the art of time management. Consistently survey your time usage methodologies, taking note of what functions admirably and what needs improvement. Embrace flexibility, being available to changing your timetable and needs as life's requests change.

Conclusion

Time usage tips for a solid way of life become the compass that guides us towards an existence of equilibrium, imperativeness, and satisfaction. Let each day become a canvas on which you balance self-care, organization, and focus as you implement these suggestions. Embrace the comprehension that using time productively isn't tied in with fitting more into your timetable yet advancing your opportunity to sustain your prosperity. The key to a life of harmony is the art of time management, where you take control of your time and live a healthy, purposeful life. Knowing that the profound power to live life to the fullest lies within the embrace of time, let the guiding principles of time management guide you toward a life of balance and limitless well-being.

7.2 Tracking down Congruity among Work and Individual Life: Embracing the Synchronized Dance of Well-Being

In the amicable quest for a satisfying presence, finding concordance among work and individual life turns into the extraordinary dance that winds around together our expert desires and individual prosperity. Like gifted accomplices on a dance floor, this fragile equilibrium permits us to lead improving lives where the two circles fit, supporting our general satisfaction and happiness. In this segment, we set out on a survey and very much made a sense of excursion to investigate the craft of tracking down concordance among work and individual life, divulging the significant force of embracing the synchronized dance of prosperity.

1. Characterize Your Boundaries

At the core of finding agreement lies the enabling demonstration of characterizing limits among work and individual life. Accept the fact that dedicating time to both aspects without allowing one to interfere with the other is essential. Put forth clear lines on working hours and focus on backing away from business related errands during individual time.

2. Focus on Your Values

Inside the domain of finding congruity lies the groundbreaking act of focusing on your qualities.

Consider what truly matters to you in your personal and professional lives. Embrace the comprehension that adjusting your everyday activities to your guiding principle cultivates a feeling of satisfaction and reason.

3. Develop Viable Time Management

In the charming quest for finding agreement, compelling using time productively turns into the core value that streamlines your everyday exercises. Make it a habit to prioritize tasks, establish attainable objectives, and devise a well-organized schedule that balances personal and professional obligations. Proficient using time productively permits you to zero in on the main thing in the two circles, cultivating a feeling of equilibrium.

4. Embrace Adaptability and Adaptability

Inside the craft of finding congruity lies the insight of embracing adaptability and flexibility. Life is dynamic, and conditions might change all of a sudden. Embrace the comprehension that being versatile permits you to explore surprising occasions and difficulties without forfeiting your prosperity.

5. Put Away Quality Time for Adored Ones

In the orchestra of tracking down concordance, sustaining your own connections turns into the endearing song that enhances your life. Put away quality time for your friends and family, whether it's family, companions, or soul mates. Embrace significant associations and value the minutes that fortify the bonds with those you care about.

6. Practice Self-Care and Mindfulness

The transformative power of self-care and mindfulness lies within the captivating realm of harmony. Rituals of self-care that rejuvenate your mind and body, like exercising, meditating, or spending time in nature, should be your top priority. To reduce stress and improve well-being, adopt mindfulness practices so that you can remain fully present and engaged in each moment.

7. Open Communication and Seeking Support

In the search for harmony, open communication becomes the key to understanding and support. Discuss transparently with your boss, associates, and friends and family about your work and individual responsibilities. Look for help from people around you, perceiving that you don't need to explore the excursion alone.

8. Observe Accomplishments and Progress

Inside the specialty of finding agreement lies the groundbreaking demonstration of praising accomplishments and progress. Recognize your accomplishments at work and in your personal life. Accept the fact that celebrating accomplishments, no matter how small, increases motivation and satisfaction.

Conclusion
 A transformative dance of defining boundaries, prioritizing values, and cultivating effective time management is required to achieve work-life balance. As you embrace this craftsmanship, let every day become a material on which you synchronize your expert yearnings with individual prosperity. Accept the fact that creating a life in which both spheres enrich and complement one another is the key to achieving harmony, not perfection. Inside the dance of finding congruence lies the way into an existence of happiness, where you nimbly balance your work and special goals. Knowing that the profound power to live life to the fullest lies within the embrace of balance, let the principles of finding harmony lead you toward a life of fulfillment and limitless well-being.

7.3 Accomplishing a Sound Balance between serious and fun activities: Embracing the Ensemble of Well-Being

In the charming ensemble of life, accomplishing a sound balance between fun and serious activities arises as the agreeable tune that sustains our expert desires and individual prosperity. We can strike a balance between our work responsibilities and the pursuit of a fulfilling life outside of work, much like skilled musicians do. In this part, we leave on a convincing excursion to investigate the craft of accomplishing a sound balance between fun and serious activities, divulging the groundbreaking force of embracing the ensemble of prosperity.

1. Set Clear Boundaries

The empowering act of setting clear boundaries is the key to achieving a healthy work-life balance. Set and adhere to specific working hours. During personal time, don't answer calls or emails about work. Accept the fact that setting limits safeguards your private life and conserves energy for leisure and relaxation.

2. Learn to Say No
The transformative wisdom of learning to say no lies within the realm of achieving balance. Be knowing about taking on extra work or responsibilities that might steer the results ominously. Embrace the force of defining your boundaries and cordially declining errands or occasions that don't line up with your quest for balance.

3. Focus on Self-Care

In the spellbinding quest for a sound balance between serious and fun activities, focusing on taking care of oneself turns into the spirit blending cadence that cultivates prosperity. Schedule time for pursuits that refuel and nourish your spirit, body, and mind. Embrace customary activity, care practices, side interests, or

investing energy with friends and family. You strengthen
your resilience and improve your capacity to overcome
obstacles at work and in life.

4. Create a Workplace with Flexibility

Promoting a flexible work environment is an essential
part of the art of finding equilibrium. Consider remote
work options or negotiating flexible work hours to
accommodate personal commitments. An adaptable
workplace engages you to adjust your timetable to line
up with your life's requests, making a more amicable
cadence.

5. Practice Care and Presence

In the spellbinding domain of accomplishing equilibrium,
care and presence become the directing stars that
anchor you right now. Mindfulness practices can help
you focus and reduce stress. Be completely present and
engaged in your work when you are at work. At the point
when you are with family or companions, be available in
those minutes without letting work contemplations
meddle.

6. Look for Support and Delegate

The empowering network of support and delegation is
part of the symphony of finding balance. When you need
it, get help from family, friends, or coworkers; remember
that you don't have to do everything on your own.

Embrace the craft of assignment, sharing errands and obligations to make additional opportunities for both work and special goals.

7. Observe Accomplishments, Large and Small

Chasing after accomplishing balance, praising accomplishments turns into the inspiring song that adds delight to your excursion. Take some time to celebrate your personal and professional accomplishments. Embrace the grasping that praising achievements, large or little, builds up your inspiration and feeling of achievement.

Conclusion

Accomplishing a sound balance between serious and fun activities is an extraordinary ensemble of defining limits, focusing on taking care of oneself, and establishing an adaptable workplace. As you embrace this art, let every day be an opportunity to combine your personal and professional goals. Embrace the comprehension that a solid balance between fun and serious activities isn't about flawlessness, yet about developing a day to day existence where both work and individual prosperity thrive. Inside the orchestra of accomplishing balance lies the way into an existence of happiness, where you nimbly explore the complexities of work and individual life. Thus, let the core values of accomplishing a solid balance between serious and fun activities lead you towards an existence of satisfaction and limitless prosperity, realizing that inside the hug of concordance lies the significant ability to carry on with life to its fullest potential.

CONTENT 8

Developing Solid Connections: Sustaining Powers of profound devotion and Connection

In the dazzling nursery of life, developing sound connections turns into the blooming substance that improves our reality with adoration, backing, and euphoria. Like gifted nursery workers, we sustain the seeds of association, permitting them to prosper into delightful bonds that hoist our prosperity and add tone to our excursion. In this part, we leave on a convincing excursion to investigate the craft of developing sound connections, revealing the groundbreaking force of watching out for the nursery of affection and association.

1. Communication and Authenticity
The empowering virtue of authenticity is central to the development of healthy relationships. Embrace the craft of being your actual self and offering your viewpoints and sentiments sincerely. Develop open and

sympathetic correspondence, making a place of refuge for significant discourse and understanding. Legitimacy and correspondence established the groundwork for trust and closeness, sustaining the underlying foundations of solid associations.

2. Undivided attention and Empathy

Inside the domain of developing solid connections lies the deep craft of undivided attention and compassion. With your full attention and presence, listen to others. Look to grasp their viewpoints, sentiments, and needs, and answer with sympathy and empathy. Undivided attention encourages profound associations and shared regard, cultivating obligations of certifiable comprehension.

3. Support and Encouragement

In the enticing endeavor of building strong relationships, encouragement and support become the sustaining rays of light that propel growth. Show up for your friends and family in the midst of hardship, offering some assistance and a listening ear. Encourage them and give them faith in their potential by celebrating their accomplishments and goals. Backing and support fortify the powers of profound devotion and care.

4. Regard Limits and Autonomy

Inside the craft of developing solid connections lies the insight regarding limits and independence. Keep in mind that everyone is unique and occupies their own space. Accept that healthy relationships allow for independence and personal development without crossing each other's boundaries.

5. Conflict Resolution with Love
 Conflict resolution becomes the harmonious rhythm that bridges differences with love and compassion in the symphony of building healthy relationships. Embrace the art of constructive conflict resolution, addressing issues with compassion and understanding. Cooperate towards settling on some mutual interest and arrangements that reinforce your security.

6. Quality Time and Shared Experiences

In the charming domain of developing sound connections, quality time and shared encounters become the captivating fortunes that make enduring recollections. Really try to invest significant energy with your friends and family, participating in exercises that cultivate association and delight. Shared encounters develop your bond and make a feeling of fellowship.

7. Celebrate and Express Gratitude

The transformative act of celebrating and expressing gratitude is part of the symphony of building healthy relationships. With your loved ones, mark milestones and accomplishments and express joy and pride in their accomplishments. Embrace the act of appreciation, communicating appreciation for the presence and cherish they bring into your life.

Conclusion: Nurturing relationships that are based on love, authenticity, and support is a transformative journey. As you embrace this art, make every day a chance to tend to the garden of connection and plant the seeds of trust, empathy, and understanding. Embrace the comprehension that sound connections require care and exertion, yet they are the blooms that advance our lives with adoration and satisfaction. Inside the hug of developing sound connections lies the way into an existence of euphoria, association, and unlimited prosperity. In this way, let the core values of affection and sympathy lead you towards a nursery of thriving connections, realizing that inside the hug of association lies the significant ability to carry on with life to its fullest potential.

8.1 Sustaining Steady Associations:

The Artful Thread That Weaves a Tapestry of Belonging, Compassion, and Strength. In the captivating fabric of life, cultivating supportive connections becomes the artful thread that weaves a tapestry. Like talented weavers, we develop connections that inspire and support us, shaping a versatile organization of affection and understanding. In this part, we set out on a convincing and drawing excursion to investigate the specialty of sustaining steady associations, disclosing the groundbreaking force of encouraging bonds that get through life's difficulties.

1. The empowering pursuit of genuine connection is at the heart of cultivating supportive connections. Seek Genuine Connection. Accept the art of building relationships based on mutual understanding and authenticity. Look for friendship with individuals who really care about your prosperity and offer your qualities, making a groundwork of trust and solace.

2. Be Available and Available

Inside the domain of sustaining strong associations lies the heartfelt act of being available and accessible for your friends and family. Accept the fact that genuine connections necessitate effort and time. Show up for them in the midst of hardship, offering a listening ear and a mindful heart. Your presence turns into an emollient that mitigates their distresses and praises their delights.

3. Offer Empathy and Understanding
 Empathy and understanding become the gentle touch that builds strong bonds in the captivating pursuit of fostering supportive connections. Put yourself in their shoes and acknowledge that their emotions and experiences are valid. Offer an empathetic hug that tells them they are in good company in their battles.

4. Celebrate Diversity and Uniqueness
 The wisdom of celebrating diversity and uniqueness lies
within the art of cultivating supportive connections.
Embrace the comprehension that every individual is
unique, with their own assets and battles. Foster an
inclusive environment where everyone feels valued and
accepted by embracing individuality.

5. Share and Support One Another's Dreams
 In the symphony of cultivating connections that are
supportive, sharing and supporting one another's
dreams becomes the harmonious melody that
encourages growth. Be truly keen on their desires and
urge them to seek after their interests. Your help turns
into a strong impetus that fills their undertakings.

6. Speak with Compassion

Inside the dazzling domain of sustaining steady
associations lies the extraordinary force of sympathetic
correspondence. Embrace the specialty of offering your
viewpoints and sentiments with consideration and
regard. Be available to share your weaknesses and
fears, making a place of refuge for fair exchange.

7. Be a Wellspring of Strength

In the orchestra of sustaining steady associations, being
a wellspring of solidarity turns into the elevating tune
that winds around strength. Help them overcome

obstacles by encouraging them and having faith in their abilities. Your unflinching help turns into an anchor that steadies them through life's tempests.

8. Support Shared Experiences

Inside the craft of sustaining strong associations lies the deep act of supporting shared encounters. Engage in activities that you both enjoy to create moments of happiness and connection. Shared encounters become esteemed recollections that extend your bond.

Conclusion

Sustaining steady associations is an extraordinary excursion of winding around an embroidery of affection, sympathy, and strength. As you embrace this workmanship, let every day become a valuable chance to cultivate profound bonds that elevate and support you. Embrace the comprehension that strong associations require sustaining and care, however they are the strings that improve our lives with adoration and strength. The key to a life of belonging, compassion, and unlimited well-being is found within the embrace of nurturing supportive connections. Thus, let the core values of genuineness and sympathy lead you towards an organization of steady associations, knowing that inside the hug of affection and understanding untruths the significant ability to carry on with life to its fullest potential.

8.2 Conveying Successfully for Positive Connections: Making the Language of Connection

In the spellbinding domain of human associations, viable correspondence turns into the sly language that winds around the texture of positive connections. Like gifted scribes, we express ourselves with care, cultivating figuring out, sympathy, and agreement. In this section, we begin a compelling journey to discover the transformative power of crafting the language of connection and the art of effectively communicating for positive relationships.

1. Tune in with Presence and Empathy

At the core of viable correspondence lies the engaging demonstration of tuning in with presence and sympathy. Accept the art of paying full attention to the speaker and appreciating their words and feelings without judging. Create a safe environment for open conversation and demonstrate empathy by attempting to comprehend their perspective and feelings.

2. Be Clear and Concise

When it comes to communicating effectively, clarity and conciseness become the guiding lights that help people understand what is being said. Offer your viewpoints and sentiments in a reasonable and clear way, staying away from equivocalness. Your messages will be more effective and easier to comprehend if you embrace the art of concise expression.

3. Use "I" Statements

In the captivating pursuit of positive relationships, the soulful practice of cultivating understanding and avoiding blame is using "I" statements. Discuss your thoughts and viewpoints utilizing "I" articulations, for example, "I feel" or "I think," rather than pointing fingers with "you" explanations. This cultivates a non-fierce climate that advances open correspondence.

4. Careful Word Selection

The art of effective communication is rooted in the wisdom of carefully selecting words. Be aware of the language you use, it is conscious and kind to guarantee it. Keep away from mockery, frightful comments, or brutal tones that might harm trust and amicability.

5. Active listening becomes the harmonious rhythm that deepens connections in the symphony of effective communication. Make eye contact, nod, and use verbal cues like "I understand" or "Tell me more" to connect with the speaker. Genuine interest and validation of the speaker's feelings are the results of active listening.

6. Be Open to Feedback

The transformative power of being open to feedback lies within the captivating realm of effective communication.

Embrace the comprehension that criticism is a chance for development and improvement. With an open mind and without getting defensive, listen to feedback to learn more about yourself and your relationships.

7. Answer, Don't React

In the ensemble of viable correspondence, answering as opposed to responding turns into the alleviating tune that diffuses strain. Pause for a minute to deal with your feelings prior to answering a circumstance, it is insightful and created to guarantee your words. Providing a gracious and poised response encourages productive discussion.

8. Keep away from Assumptions

Inside the specialty of powerful correspondence lies the insight of keeping away from suspicions. Request explanation when required, as opposed to making presumptions about others' viewpoints or expectations. This forestalls errors and advances clearness in correspondence.

Conclusion
 Creating the language of connection, embracing active listening, empathy, and clarity are the transformative steps in effectively communicating for positive relationships. As you embrace this workmanship, let every discussion become a chance to sustain understanding and congruity. Accept that while loving

and compassionate language enriches our relationships, effective communication is a skill that requires practice and mindfulness. Inside the hug of imparting successfully for positive connections lies the way into an existence of significant associations, sympathy, and endless prosperity. Knowing that the profound power to live life to the fullest lies within the language of connection, let the guiding principles of active listening and thoughtful expression lead you toward a world of positive relationships.

8.3 Managing Disagreement Using Compassion and Respect: Exploring the Oceans of Conflict with Grace

In the turbulent oceans of human communications, taking care of contention with sympathy and regard arises as the compass that guides us through difficult situations. Like gifted mariners, we explore conflicts with understanding and effortlessness, cultivating goal and congruence. In this segment, we leave on a surveying excursion to investigate the craft of taking care of contention with sympathy and regard, divulging the extraordinary force of embracing empathy in the midst of strife.

1. Cultivate Empathy
The empowering practice of cultivating empathy is at the heart of handling conflict with empathy and respect. Even when there are disagreements, try to comprehend

other people's feelings and points of view. Put yourself in their shoes and show compassion for their emotions and experiences. In times of conflict, empathy builds a bridge of understanding.

2. Tune in with Openness

Inside the domain of taking care of contention, tuning in with receptiveness turns into the core value that cultivates useful discourse. Put away your predispositions and inclinations, permitting the other individual to offer their viewpoints and sentiments without interference. Open listening confirms their experiences and opens the door to mutual understanding.

3. Express Yourself Thoughtfully

In the enamoring quest for settling struggle with sympathy and regard, expressing yourself nicely turns into the profound craftsmanship that advances sound correspondence. Try not to utilize harmful or forceful language that might raise strains. Instead, be calm and respectful when expressing your thoughts and concerns, encouraging productive conversation.

4. Center around Arrangements, Not Blame

Inside the craft of dealing with struggle lies the insight of zeroing in on arrangements as opposed to finding fault. Find solutions that address the fundamental issues by working together with the other person. Embrace the comprehension that contention is a chance for development and learning, and together, you can make progress toward a goal that fulfills the two players.

5. Take Responsibility for Your Actions

In the symphony of conflict management, taking responsibility for your actions becomes the harmonies that encourage accountability. Recognize your part in the contention and apologize if fundamental. Recognize the ways in which your actions may have contributed to the disagreement and practice the art of self-reflection.

6. Remain Calm and Composed

Remaining calm and composed becomes the transformative force that reduces tensions in the captivating field of conflict management. Avoid reactivity that could aggravate the situation and embrace emotional regulation. Keeping a feeling of quiet considers objective conversation and critical thinking.

7. Look for Normal Ground

In the orchestra of taking care of contention with sympathy and regard, looking for shared view turns into the amicable musicality that brings goal. Use areas of agreement or common interests as a starting point to build on. Embrace compromise while essential, perceiving that figuring out some shared interest encourages agreement.

8. Know When to Take a Break

 The wisdom of knowing when to take a break is part of the art of conflict resolution. It is acceptable to temporarily withdraw from the situation to calm down if feelings are running high. Refocusing takes into consideration a new viewpoint and an opportunity to move toward the contention with restored compassion and understanding.

Conclusion] A transformative journey of embracing compassion and understanding in the face of discord is handling conflict with empathy and respect. Let every conflict become an opportunity to navigate with grace, empathy, and openness as you review these principles. Embrace the comprehension that settling clashes with compassion reinforces connections and advances an agreeable presence. Inside the hug of taking care of contention with sympathy and regard lies the way into an existence of solid correspondence, development, and limitless prosperity. Knowing that the profound power to navigate life's challenges with grace and compassion lies within the art of conflict management, allow the guiding principles of empathy and respect to lead you toward smoother waters.

CONTENT 9

Solid Propensities for the Brain and Soul:

Healthy Habits Bloom as the Vibrant Flowers that Nurture Our Inner Well-being and Bring Joy to Our Lives in the Enchanting Sanctuary of Our Minds and Souls. Like committed guardians, we keep an eye on these propensities, cultivating an amicable relationship with ourselves and our general surroundings. In this segment, we leave on a convincing and drawing excursion to investigate the craft of developing solid propensities for the psyche and soul, divulging the extraordinary force of taking care of oneself and development.

1. Develop Mindfulness

At the core of solid propensities for the brain and soul lies the engaging act of developing care. Embrace the specialty of being completely present in every second, without judgment. Savor the sights, sounds, and sensations around you by engaging your senses. You can live your life with more clarity and serenity by practicing mindfulness, which helps you cultivate inner peace and reduce stress.

2. Embrace Gratitude

When it comes to healthy habits, embracing gratitude becomes the lighthouse that guides our days filled with joy and appreciation. Make time every day to appreciate the good things in your life and the blessings you have received. Accept the knowledge that expressing gratitude changes your perspective and opens your heart to the abundance around you.

3. Practice Self-Compassion

Self-compassion becomes the soulful embrace that nourishes our self-worth in the captivating pursuit of healthy habits for the mind and soul. Indulge yourself with a similar benevolence and understanding you would offer a dear companion. Embrace self-sympathy in the midst of trouble, perceiving that everybody faces difficulties, and it's OK to be delicate with yourself.

4. Participate in Imaginative Expression

Inside the craft of developing sound propensities lies the extraordinary force of imaginative articulation. Investigate exercises that permit your spirit to take off, whether it's composition, painting, moving, or playing an instrument. Taking part in imaginative articulation encourages a feeling of satisfaction and interfaces you with your bona fide self.

5. Focus on Rest and Relaxation

In the ensemble of solid propensities, focusing on rest and unwinding turns into the amicable musicality that revives your psyche and soul. Embrace the specialty of dialing back, permitting yourself to rest when required. Practice unwinding strategies, like reflection or profound breathing, to deliver pressure and advance internal harmony.

6. Find Meaningful Connections
In the enticing world of healthy habits, finding meaningful connections transforms into the heart-warming melody that nourishes our souls. Be surrounded by people who lift you up and help you. Develop bona fide connections that permit you to share your delights and weaknesses, cultivating a feeling of having a place and love.

7. Set Individual Boundaries

In the ensemble of sound propensities for the brain and soul, defining individual limits turns into the engaging harmony that protects your prosperity. Embrace the specialty of saying "no" while important, safeguarding your significant investment. You can prioritize self-care and keep your life in balance by setting boundaries.

8. Embrace Lifelong Learning

The wisdom of embracing lifelong learning lies within the art of developing healthy habits. Participate in exercises that animate your psyche and extend your viewpoints. Attend workshops, read books, or take up hobbies that pique your interest. Personal development and a sense of purpose are facilitated by embracing lifelong learning.

Conclusion

Sound propensities for the brain and soul are the extraordinary blossoms that advance our lives with care, appreciation, and self-empathy. As you embrace these propensities, let every day become a potential chance to watch out for the nursery of your internal safe-haven, supporting taking care of oneself and development. Accept that developing healthy habits is a journey of self-discovery and evolution rather than a destination. Inside the hug of solid propensities for the psyche and soul lies the way into an existence of inward congruity, satisfaction, and endless prosperity. In this way, let the core values of care and self-sympathy lead you towards a universe of thriving propensities, realizing that inside the craft of taking care of oneself lies the significant influence to sustain your brain and soul, improving your reality with affection, harmony, and essentialness.

9.1 Meditation and mindfulness practices: Beginning a Journey of Inner Peace

The practice of mindfulness and meditation shines like a shining beacon in the realm of self-discovery and inner peace, leading us to a profound connection with our true selves. We set out on a journey of stillness and awareness, like patient explorers, to unravel the depths of our consciousness and find solace in the whirlwinds of life. In this segment, we dig into the checking on process, investigating the groundbreaking force of rehearsing care and reflection and its effect on our general prosperity.

1. Embracing the Present Moment

At the center of care and contemplation lies the enabling demonstration of embracing the current second. Through careful mindfulness, we tune into the lavishness of our encounters, turning out to be completely drenched in every breath, sensation, and thought. We can let go of worries about the past or the future with this increased presence, cultivating a sense of calm and acceptance.

2. Developing Inward Stillness

Inside the domain of care and reflection, developing inward quietness turns into the peaceful desert spring that re-energizes our brains and spirits. Through committed practice, we figure out how to calm the ceaseless prattle of our brains, tracking down asylum in the immense breadth of tranquility inside. During times of stress, this inner calm serves as a haven and provides clarity for making decisions.

3. Supporting Self-Compassion

In the enamoring quest for care and contemplation, self-sympathy turns into the heartfelt hug that recuperates our internal injuries. As we become mindful of our viewpoints and feelings without judgment, we figure out how to stretch out generosity and understanding to ourselves. Self-sympathy turns into an emollient that relieves self-analysis and encourages a caring relationship with our own being.

4. Upgrading Close to home Regulation

Inside the craft of rehearsing care and contemplation lies the extraordinary force of improving close to home guidelines. Through careful perception, we foster the ability to recognize our feelings without becoming snared in them. This capacity to understand individuals on a profound level permits us to answer testing circumstances with more noteworthy poise and shrewdness.

5. Developing Appreciation and Joy

In the orchestra of care and reflection, developing appreciation and bliss turns into the amicable tune that improves our lives with energy. As we notice existence with care, we perceive the overflow of endowments that encompass us. Appreciation turns into a characteristic articulation, mixing our hearts with a significant feeling of euphoria and happiness.

6. The soul-stirring practice of fostering resilience can be found within the captivating realms of mindfulness and meditation. As we fabricate a groundwork of internal harmony, we become better prepared to explore life's inescapable difficulties. In times of turbulence, mindfulness serves as an anchor that keeps us grounded and enables us to bounce back with strength and adaptability.

7. Extending Compassion and Connection

In the ensemble of care and reflection, extending sympathy and association become the endearing notes that span the holes among us and others. We can become more sensitive to the feelings and experiences of those around us by practicing mindful awareness. This elevated compassion encourages certified associations, making a feeling of unity with every single living being.

8. Developing Self-Awareness

Inside the craft of rehearsing care and reflection lies the insight of developing mindfulness. Without attachment, we gain insight into our subconscious beliefs and conditioning by observing our thoughts and patterns.

This mindfulness turns into an impetus for self-improvement and change.

Conclusion

Rehearsing care and reflection is an extraordinary excursion of self-disclosure, internal peacefulness, and extended cognizance. As we survey the effect of these practices, let every second turn into a chance to be completely present and embrace the quietness inside. Accept the fact that mindfulness and meditation are not just tools; rather, they open the door to profound self-awareness and authentic connection to the world. Inside the hug of care and contemplation lies the way into an existence of harmony, clearness, and endless prosperity. Thus, let the core values of care and self-empathy lead you towards a universe of internal congruity, realizing that inside the craft of reflection lies the significant ability to support your psyche and soul, enabling you to explore life's excursion with elegance and intelligence.

9.2 Participating in Imaginative Pursuits: Unleashing the Colorful Symphony That Is Within

When we engage in creative pursuits, our existence is transformed into a vibrant palette that is infused with hues of imagination, expression, and joy. Like trying specialists, we embrace the opportunity to make, releasing the bright orchestra inside us and painting an embroidery of self-disclosure and satisfaction. In this part, we leave on a convincing and drawing excursion to investigate the groundbreaking force of taking part in imaginative pursuits, disentangling the significant effect it has on our prosperity and development.

1. Embracing Self-Expression

At the core of taking part in imaginative pursuits lies the engaging demonstration of embracing self-articulation. Through different creative outlets like work of art, composing, moving, or making, we track down the mental fortitude to convey our considerations, feelings, and points of view. This unrestricted self-expression transforms into a liberating journey of authenticity and self-discovery.

2. Developing Stream and Mindfulness

Inside the domain of imaginative pursuits, developing stream and care turns into the core value that drenches us right now. Time seems to disappear as we engage in creative pursuits, and we enter a state of flow, or total concentration on the task at hand. This flow transforms into a meditative experience that cultivates calm and mindfulness.

3. Opening Creative mind and Innovation

In the dazzling quest for inventive pursuits, opening creative minds and advancement turns into the spirit blending tune that extends the limits of what is conceivable. Through craftsmanship, we rise above constraints and embrace unfathomable imagination. This creative investigation advances our imaginative undertakings as well as energizes development in different parts of life.

4. Taking Care of One's Emotions
 The wisdom of taking care of one's emotions lies within the practice of engaging in creative pursuits. Imaginative articulation turns into a restorative outlet, permitting us to process and deliver feelings in a solid manner. Whether it's writing in a diary, playing music, or making visual workmanship, the demonstration of making turns into a recuperating salve for our souls.

5. Building Resilience and Adaptability
In the symphony of creative endeavors, developing one's resilience and adaptability becomes the harmonious rhythm that bolsters one's spirit. We embrace the courage to face challenges and uncertainties as we experiment with various art forms. This eagerness to investigate and adjust cultivates strength despite life's promising and less promising times.

6. Fostering Connection and Collaboration
The transformative power of fostering connection and collaboration lies within the captivating realm of creative endeavors. Taking part in imaginative exercises with others encourages brotherhood and a feeling of having a place. When people work together on art projects, the

end result is a beautiful example of unity and a common goal.

7. Empowering Energy and Joy

In the ensemble of imaginative pursuits, empowering perkiness and euphoria turns into the endearing notes that jazz up our spirits. Inventiveness welcomes us to be perky and unconstrained, reviving the innocent miracle inside. This cheerful investigation turns into a festival of life's straightforward delights.

8. Engaging Individual Growth

Inside the specialty of taking part in imaginative pursuits lies the insight of engaging self-improvement. As we focus on the excursion of creation, we experience provokes that welcome us to learn and develop. The course of creation turns into an extraordinary way of constant development and self-disclosure.

Conclusion

Taking part in imaginative pursuits is a groundbreaking excursion of self-articulation, care, and development. Begin this journey by making every brushstroke, dance step, and word you write an opportunity to bring out the vibrant symphony that is already within you. Embrace the comprehension that imagination isn't an ability held for a chosen handful however an inheritance of each and every spirit. Inside the hug of innovative pursuits lies the way into an existence of self-disclosure, bliss, and vast prosperity. In light of the fact that the profound power to paint a life of authenticity and fulfillment lies within the canvas of creativity, allow the guiding principles of self-expression and playfulness to lead you toward a world of vibrant imagination.

9.3 Embracing Appreciation and Positive Reasoning:

Embracing gratitude and positive thinking emerge as the radiant thread that weaves a tapestry of joy, abundance, and resilience in the tapestry of our thoughts and emotions.

We cultivate the seeds of gratitude and optimism, transforming our outlook on life and arousing a profound appreciation for the present moment, like mental alchemists. In this segment, we dive into the extraordinary force of embracing appreciation and positive reasoning, enlightening the way to a seriously satisfying and brilliant presence.

1. The Specialty of Gratitude

At the core of embracing appreciation lies the engaging specialty of recognizing the endowments that encompass us. It is the craft of counting our gifts, of all shapes and sizes, and communicating appreciation for the excellence of life. Appreciation moves our concentration from what we need to what we have,

mixing our days with a feeling of overflow and
happiness.

2. Releasing the Force of Positive Thinking

Inside the domain of positive reasoning falsehoods the
extraordinary ability to shape our existence. Our
contemplations hold the way into our encounters, and by
developing a positive mentality, we open ways to
conceivable outcomes and valuable open doors.
Positive reasoning enables us to beat difficulties with
strength and find arrangements where others see
impediments.

3. The Far reaching influence of Positivity

In the dazzling quest for embracing appreciation and
positive reasoning, we reveal the far reaching influence
that these practices have on our lives and people
around us. Others are inspired and encouraged when
we radiate positivity into the world. Our local
communities and the entire world are impacted by the
positive ripple that extends beyond our immediate
vicinity.

4. Finding Beauty in the Present Moment
 The wisdom of finding beauty in the present moment
can be found in the art of gratitude and positive thinking.
It's the art of savoring the little pleasures in life, like a
warm hug, a stunning sunset, or a sincere conversation.

By being available and careful, we open the significant magnificence concealed in regular encounters.

5. Developing a Versatile Spirit

In the ensemble of embracing appreciation and positive reasoning, we find the agreeable cadence of developing a tough soul. We develop the inner strength to overcome obstacles and disappointments when we approach them with optimism. Appreciation turns into the anchor that steadies us in the midst of life's tempests.

6. Sustaining Self-Compassion

Inside the dazzling domain of appreciation and positive reasoning falsehoods the extraordinary force of supporting self-sympathy. Self-love and acceptance are cultivated as we embrace gratitude for our distinctive qualities and achievements. Positive reasoning turns into a sustaining voice that urges us to be kinder to ourselves, cultivating a caring relationship with our own being.

7. The Heartwarming Notes of Joy that Come from Giving and Sharing.
We discover the heartwarming notes of joy that come from giving and sharing in the symphony of positive thinking and gratitude. Appreciation propels us to stretch out consideration to other people, and positive reasoning constrains us to rouse and uphold everyone

around us. The delight of giving turns into a sincere
dance of correspondence and association.

8. Creating an Upward Spiral of Well-Being
The wisdom of creating an upward spiral of well-being
lies within the art of embracing gratitude and positive
thinking. As we feed our brains with energy, it turns into
a self-sustaining cycle that draws in additional
endowments and valuable open doors into our lives.
Positive thinking and showing gratitude lead to new
beginnings and a brighter future.

Conclusion

Embracing appreciation and positive reasoning is a
groundbreaking excursion of enlivening to the overflow
of life and supporting a brilliant outlook. Let each day
become an opportunity to cultivate gratitude and
optimism in your heart as you embrace these practices.
Embrace the comprehension that appreciation and
positive reasoning are not brief feelings but rather strong
decisions that shape our world. Inside the hug of
appreciation and positive reasoning untruths the way
into an existence of bliss, strength, and limitless
prosperity. Knowing that the profound power to paint
your life with a palette of abundance and serenity lies
within the art of gratitude and positive thinking, allow the
guiding principles of appreciation and optimism to lead
you toward a world of radiant living.

CONTENT 10

Beating Difficulties and Misfortunes: Fashioning Strength Despite Adversity

In the embroidered artwork of life, difficulties and misfortunes are the multifaceted bunches that test the strength of our determination and character. Like daring fighters, we walk forward, confronting difficulty with steady assurance and fortitude. In this section, we embark on a compelling and interesting journey to discover the indomitable spirit that emerges from struggle and the transformative power of overcoming obstacles.

1. Embracing the Journey of Growth
 The empowering act of embracing the journey of growth is at the heart of overcoming obstacles and setbacks. Challenges become impetus for change, welcoming us to develop and grow past our usual ranges of familiarity. We discover new strengths and abilities within ourselves with each obstacle we overcome.

2. Cultivating Resilience and Adaptability
 The transformative power of cultivating resilience and adaptability lies within the realm of overcoming challenges. Like the strong oak that curves with the breeze, versatility permits us to endure life's tempests without breaking. We figure out how to adjust to always evolving conditions, tracking down savvy fixes to explore through unfamiliar areas.

3. Transforming Mishaps into Venturing Stones

In the enthralling quest for defeating mishaps, we reveal the heartfelt specialty of transforming misfortunes into venturing stones. Rather than surrendering to overcome, we consider mishaps to be open doors for learning and development. Every difficulty turns into a significant example that pushes us forward on our way to progress.

4. Tackling the Force of Perseverance

Inside the specialty of beating difficulties lies the insight of saddling the force of diligence. When confronted with impediments, we gather our inward strength and assurance to continue to push ahead. Steadiness turns into the reference point that lights our direction through the haziest of times.

5. Tracking down Help in Community

In the ensemble of conquering difficulties and mishaps, we find the amicable musicality of tracking down help in the local area. Encircling ourselves with an organization of understanding and caring people gives solace and consolation during troublesome times. Knowing that we are not on our own journey, we share our difficulties and celebrate our successes together.

6. Cultivating a Positive Mindset
 We discover the transformative power of cultivating a positive mindset within the captivating field of overcoming obstacles. We shift our focus from issues to possibilities as we embrace optimism. A positive outlook enables us to move toward difficulties with certainty and innovativeness.

7. Learning from Setbacks
 The uplifting notes of development and learning can be heard in the symphony of overcoming obstacles. Every misfortune turns into a chance to reflect and acquire insight. By embracing the examples concealed inside difficulties, we become better prepared to confront future obstructions.

8. Observing Strength and Triumph

Inside the craft of defeating difficulties and misfortunes lies the insight of commending versatility and win. No matter how insignificant the victory, it becomes evidence of our strength and perseverance. Commending our versatility helps us to remember the unstoppable soul that dwells inside us.

Conclusion

Conquering difficulties and mishaps is a groundbreaking excursion of strength, development, and win. Allow each moment to serve as an opportunity to triumph over adversity with bravery and determination as you navigate life's challenges. Accept that difficulties are actually steps on the way to greatness rather than obstacles. Inside the hug of beating difficulties and misfortunes lies the way into an existence of unfaltering strength, determination, and endless prosperity. Recognizing that the profound power to forge your destiny with resilience and triumph lies within the art of overcoming challenges, allow the guiding principles of adaptability and resilience to lead you toward a world of triumph and growth.

10.1 Versatility Even with Affliction: Immovable Strength In the midst of Life's Trials

In the theater of life, strength remains as the immovable hero, sparkling splendidly in the midst of the shadows of misfortune. We use our resilience to overcome obstacles with unwavering strength and courage, like a phoenix rising from the ashes. In this part, we set out on a convincing and engaging excursion to investigate the extraordinary force of strength, uncovering the unstoppable soul that rises out of the cauldron of life's preliminaries.

1. Embracing the Power of Adaptability
The empowering act of embracing the power of adaptability is at the heart of resilience. Life's difficulties frequently present startling exciting bends in the road, requesting us to change our sails in new bearings. We are able to adapt to the forces of change through resilience, turning challenges into opportunities for development.

2. Sustaining Internal Strength and Courage

Inside the domain of flexibility stands the groundbreaking force of sustaining internal strength and boldness. Adversity puts us to the test at the core of who we are, revealing strengths we may not have known we possessed. Through strength, we draw from this inward repository of mental fortitude, tracking down the dauntlessness to confront our feelings of trepidation and defeated obstructions.

3. Transforming Difficulties into Venturing Stones

In the enamoring quest for strength, we reveal the deep craft of transforming misfortunes into venturing stones. We don't let setbacks define us; rather, we view them as valuable learning opportunities. We can rise from the ashes of disappointment and forge ahead with

newfound wisdom and determination when we have
resilience.

4. Tracking down Silver Linings in Adversity

Inside the craft of versatility lies the insight of tracking
down silver linings in affliction. There are lessons to be
learned and glimmerings of hope to be found even in the
worst of times. Strength empowers us to search out the
up-sides, zeroing in on what we have some control over
as opposed to harping on what is outside our ability to
understand.

5. Embracing Self-Compassion

In the ensemble of versatility, we find the amicable beat
of embracing self-empathy. Resilience reminds us to be
kind to ourselves in the face of difficulties and
acknowledges that we are only human. Embracing
self-empathy sustains our close to home prosperity and
encourages a caring relationship with ourselves.

6. Drawing Backing from Community

Inside the dazzling domain of versatility, we track down
the inspiring notes of drawing support from the local
area. When we rely on the understanding and support of
those around us, our resilience gains strength. Together,
we endure the hardships of life, realizing that we are in
good company on our excursion.

7. Cultivating a Growth Mindset
We discover the transformative power of cultivating a growth mindset in the symphony of resilience. Strength welcomes us to consider difficulties to be open doors for learning and development. With a development outlook, we approach hindrances with interest and assurance, realizing that progress comes from embracing the interaction.

8. Celebrating Victory Over Adversity
The wisdom of celebrating victory over adversity is a part of the art of resilience. We acknowledge our inherent strength each time we triumph over difficulties. Resilience is celebrated because it reinforces our self-confidence and confidence in our ability to deal with life's challenges.

Conclusion

Versatility notwithstanding misfortune is an extraordinary excursion of flexibility, inward strength, and win. As you explore through life's preliminaries, let every second turn into a chance to saddle the force of flexibility. Accept that resilience is a skill that can be developed and honed through life's experiences rather than a fixed trait. Inside the hug of versatility lies the way into an existence of unflinching strength, boldness, and vast prosperity. Thus, let the core values of versatility and self-empathy lead you towards a universe of win and development, realizing that inside the specialty of flexibility lies the significant ability to transcend life's difficulties with elegance and resolute strength.

10.2 Coming Through Obstacles: Resilience as the Art of Rebounding

In the symphony of life, setbacks are the unanticipated notes that challenge our melody. However, resilience becomes the conductor, directing us to bounce back with a newfound strength and determination. We embrace the art of rebounding from setbacks, weaving a captivating tale of resilience and triumph like a ballerina gracefully rising from a fall. In this segment, we set out on a convincing and connecting with excursion to investigate the extraordinary force of returning from difficulties, disclosing the unstoppable soul that rises up out of the cauldron of misfortune.

1. Embracing the Journey of Resilience
 The empowering act of embracing the journey of resilience is at the heart of recovering from setbacks. It is the comprehension that mishaps are not impasses however simple diversions on our way to progress. Strength enables us to ascend with boldness and conviction, realizing that each difficulty is a chance for development and change.

2. Transforming Affliction into Opportunity

Inside the domain of returning from mishaps, we find the extraordinary force of transforming difficulty into a potential open door. Every difficulty turns into a fresh start, welcoming us to illustrate probability and progress. Versatility permits us to consider mishaps to be impetus for change, driving us towards strange skylines.

3. Cultivating a Positive Mindset
We discover the soulful art of cultivating a positive mindset in the captivating pursuit of recovery. We are encouraged to challenge negative thoughts and replace them with affirmations that give us strength through resilience. A positive mentality turns into the springboard that impels us forward with good faith and assurance.

4. Bridling the Force of Perseverance

Inside the craft of returning from difficulties lies the insight of bridling the force of steadiness. We summon our unwavering spirit to persevere in our efforts when confronted with difficulties. Determination turns into the consistent musicality that brings us through obstructions, preparing to win.

5. Looking for Help and Encouragement

In the ensemble of quickly returning from mishaps, we find the agreeable mood of looking for help and consolation. We are reminded by resilience that we are not alone in dealing with setbacks. Our resolve is strengthened and invaluable guidance is provided when we surround ourselves with a supportive network of family, friends, or mentors.

6. Gaining and Developing from Setbacks

Inside the enamoring domain of returning, we track down the endearing notes of learning and development. Every difficulty turns into a homeroom where we gain shrewdness and understanding. We can use setbacks as opportunities for self-discovery and gain wisdom and strength from them through resilience.

7. Embracing Flexibility and Adaptability
We discover the transformative power of embracing flexibility and adaptability in the symphony of resilience. We must be willing to change our approach and open to change in order to recover from setbacks. Versatility permits us to stream with life's ebbs and flows, embracing the excellence of advancement smoothly.

8. Observing Victory over Setbacks

Inside the craft of returning falsehoods the insight of celebrating win over misfortunes. We celebrate our resilience and development each time we overcome adversity. Celebrating win turns into a sign of our ability to survive, persuading us to confront future difficulties with certainty and assurance.

Conclusion

Returning from misfortunes is a groundbreaking excursion of strength, flexibility, and win. As you explore through life's diversions, let every second turn into a chance to bounce back with mental fortitude and unflinching strength. Embrace the comprehension that difficulties are not routs, however venturing stones on the way to progress. Inside the hug of returning falsehoods the way into an existence of development, win, and vast prosperity. Therefore, allow the principles of perseverance and positivity to guide you toward a world of resilience and success, knowing that the profound power to rise above setbacks with grace and unwavering strength lies within the art of rebounding.

10.3 Looking for Proficient Help When Required:

The Beacon of Hope That Illuminates the Path to Healing and Growth. In the tapestry of life, there are times when the burdens become too heavy to bear on one's own, and seeking professional support becomes the beacon of hope. Professional support empowers us to overcome obstacles with newfound clarity and strength, like a compass that guides us through the complexities of our emotions and challenges. In this part, we set out on a convincing and connecting excursion to investigate the extraordinary force of looking for proficient help while required, uncovering the significant effect it can have on our prosperity and self-awareness.

1. Embracing the Courage to Reach Out

The empowering act of embracing the courage to reach out is at the heart of seeking professional support. The comprehension of looking for help is definitely not an indication of shortcoming yet a demonstration of our solidarity and mindfulness. By connecting with experts, we honor our excursion towards development and mending.

2. Making a Safe and Sustaining Space

Inside the domain of expert help, we track down the groundbreaking force of making a safe and sustaining space. This space turns into a safe-haven where we can put ourselves out there straightforwardly and without judgment. It permits us to investigate our contemplations and feelings, preparing for self-revelation and mending.

3. Acquiring New Points of view and Insights

In the dazzling quest for proficient help, we uncover the heartfelt craft of acquiring new points of view and experiences. Professionals with training shed new light on our problems and provide valuable insights that we may have missed. These new points of view become impetus for development and change.

4. Healing Emotional Wounds
The wisdom of healing emotional wounds lies within the art of seeking professional support. We are guided

through the process of acknowledging and processing our emotions by trained counselors or therapists. A transformative path to inner peace and emotional well-being emerges from this therapeutic journey.

5. Exploring Life Transitions

In the ensemble of looking for proficient help, we find the agreeable musicality of exploring life advances. Professionals offer support during times of uncertainty, whether it's a major life decision, a career shift, or a loss. Their mastery turns into a directing light, engaging us to go with informed decisions.

6. Building Adapting Abilities and Resilience

Inside the enamoring domain of looking for proficient help, we track down the inspiring notes of building adapting abilities and strength. Experts furnish us with viable apparatuses to adapt to pressure, tension, or testing circumstances. As we navigate life's ups and downs, these skills become valuable assets.

7. Developing Self-Compassion

In the orchestra of expert help, we uncover the extraordinary force of developing self-sympathy. We learn to be gentle with ourselves through therapy or counseling, accepting the realization that we are all human and deserving of kindness. Self-empathy turns into the sustaining embrace that cultivates a sound connection with ourselves.

8. Engaging Self-awareness

Inside the specialty of looking for proficient help lies the insight of engaging self-awareness. As we leave on this excursion, we perceive the groundbreaking effect it can have on our lives. Looking for proficient help turns into a strong step towards turning into our best selves.

Conclusion: A transformative journey of healing, development, and empowerment begins when you seek professional assistance when you need it. As you explore through life's difficulties, let every second turn into a chance to connect for direction and backing. Embrace the comprehension that looking for help is a gutsy demonstration that makes you ready for self-improvement and prosperity. Inside the hug of expert help lies the way into an existence of recuperating, strength, and vast development. In this way, let the core values of boldness and self-sympathy lead you towards a universe of strengthening and change, realizing that inside the craft of looking for proficient help lies the significant ability to recuperate and prosper with unfaltering strength.

CONTENT 11

Sustainability in the Long Run:

Long-term sustainability emerges as the harmonious melody that orchestrates a flourishing future for our planet and its inhabitants in the symphony of existence. We accept our responsibility to safeguard our society, economy, and environment as compassionate stewards in order to leave a legacy of prosperity for future generations. In this segment, we set out on a convincing and connecting tour to investigate the extraordinary force of long haul maintainability, disclosing the significant effect it can have on our reality and the heritage we abandon.

1. Embracing the Vision of a Flourishing Future
 The empowering act of embracing the vision of a thriving future is at the heart of long-term sustainability. It is the awareness that the world we leave for our children

and future generations is shaped by our actions today. Long haul supportability turns into the directing compass that adjusts our choices to the aggregate prosperity of our planet.

2. Encouraging Natural Stewardship

Inside the domain of long haul maintainability, we track down the groundbreaking force of encouraging ecological stewardship. We become conscious of our impact on the environment when we acknowledge the interconnectedness of all life. Stewardship turns into a promise to save assets, diminish squander, and safeguard the normal world for people in the future.

3. Making Tough and Comprehensive Societies

In the enrapturing quest for long haul supportability, we reveal the deep specialty of making versatile and comprehensive social orders. Maintainability goes past natural worries and stretches out to social value and equity. By tending to disparities and cultivating inclusivity, we make ready for social orders that flourish together, abandoning nobody.

4. Nurturing Responsible Economic Practices

 The wisdom of cultivating responsible economic practices is entwined with the art of long-term sustainability. Profits as well as the impact on society and the environment are priorities for sustainable businesses. By embracing roundabout economy models, organizations limit squander and focus on asset proficiency, adding to a maintainable future.

5. Preserving Biodiversity and Ecosystems
 The harmonious rhythm of preserving biodiversity and ecosystems is discovered in the symphony of long-term sustainability. Every species assumes a remarkable part in the trap of life, and preservation endeavors become a demonstration of our interconnectedness. We ensure our planet's health and resilience by safeguarding ecosystems.

6. Putting resources into Sustainable Energy

Inside the enamoring domain of long haul manageability, we track down the endearing notes of putting resources into sustainable power. We can combat climate change and reduce greenhouse gas emissions by switching to clean, renewable sources. As the energy of the future, renewable energy will ensure a healthy and sustainable planet.

7. Instructing and Enabling Future Generations

In the orchestra of long haul manageability, we reveal the groundbreaking force of teaching and engaging people in the future. By outfitting youngsters with information about maintainability and natural stewardship, we plant seeds for a fate of cognizant navigation and capable activity.

8. Embracing Advancement and Technology

Inside the craft of long haul maintainability lies the insight of embracing development and innovation. From climate adaptation to effective waste management, scientific and technological advancements offer solutions to global issues. We move toward a sustainable future as a result of innovation becoming a driving force.

Conclusion

Long-term sustainability is a transformative journey that requires stewardship, responsibility, and imaginative thinking. As we explore through the intricacies of our reality, let every second turn into a chance to add to a prospering future. Accept that sustainability is not a distant objective but rather a way of life that begins with conscious choices made today. Inside the hug of long haul manageability lies the way into a universe of overflow, concordance, and endless prosperity for a long time into the future. In this way, let the core values of natural stewardship and development lead you towards a universe of supportability and heritage, realizing that inside the craft of long haul manageability lies the significant ability to make a thriving future that resounds through the ages.

11.1 Making Sound Living a Long lasting Excursion:

Making healthy living a journey that lasts a lifetime becomes the vibrant thread that weaves a story of vitality, happiness, and fulfillment in the grand tapestry of life. Wellness empowers us to savor the beauty of each moment and thrive in mind, body, and soul, like a faithful companion who walks alongside us through every chapter. In this section, we set out on a compelling and interesting journey to learn about the profound impact that making healthy living a lifelong commitment has on our overall well-being and enthusiasm for life.

1. Embracing All encompassing Wellness

At the core of making sound living a long lasting excursion lies the engaging demonstration of embracing all encompassing wellbeing. The realization that true well-being encompasses mental, emotional, and spiritual equilibrium in addition to physical health. The compass that directs us toward a life that is both harmonious and satisfying is holistic wellness.

2. The transformative power of cultivating healthy habits is found within the context of lifelong wellness. These propensities become the structure blocks of our prosperity, from nutritious eating and ordinary activity to care and taking care of oneself. Embracing sound propensities makes way for an existence of essentialness and strength.

3. Embracing Mindful Living

We discover the soulful art of embracing mindful living in the captivating pursuit of lifelong wellness. Care turns into the key that opens the wealth of every second, permitting us to be completely present and relish life's delights. With careful mindfulness, we develop a more profound association with ourselves and our general surroundings.

4. Cultivating Deep rooted Learning

Inside the craft of deep rooted wellbeing lies the insight of cultivating long lasting learning. As we venture through life, we embrace the interest to grow our insight and investigate new skylines. Deep rooted learning turns into the fuel that lights our interests and keeps our psyches dynamic and locked in.

5. Prioritizing Self-Care
We discover the harmonious rhythm of prioritizing self-care in the symphony of lifelong wellness. Taking care of oneself turns into the delicate touch that feeds our spirits and renews our energy. We build a foundation of well-being that lasts throughout our lives by scheduling time for rest, relaxation, and enjoyable activities.

6. Cultivating Meaningful Connections

We find the warm notes of cultivating meaningful connections within the captivating realm of lifelong wellness. Positive connections become mainstays of help and wellsprings of satisfaction. As we sustain veritable associations with others, we make a feeling of having a place and close to home prosperity.

7. Embracing Resilience and Adaptability
We discover the transformative power of embracing resilience and adaptability in the symphony of lifelong wellness. Life gives us difficulties and changes, however with versatility, we return quickly from mishaps and move forward with strength. We are able to move with the currents of life and find grace in every season when we embrace adaptability.

8. Celebrating the Journey

The wisdom of celebrating the journey itself lies within the art of making healthy living a lifelong journey. In our pursuit of happiness, each day becomes a milestone. By commending our advancement, regardless of how little, we honor the responsibility we make to ourselves and set up to proceed with development and satisfaction.

Conclusion
Making healthy living a journey that lasts a lifetime is a life-changing commitment to happiness, growth, and wellness. Let each moment serve as an opportunity to embrace well-being and self-discovery as you move through life's chapters. Embrace the comprehension that deep rooted wellbeing isn't a location yet a wonderful excursion of constant development and taking care of oneself. The key to a life of vitality, contentment, and

limitless well-being lies within the embrace of making healthy living a journey that lasts a lifetime. In this way, let the core values of comprehensive wellbeing and versatility lead you towards a universe of long lasting essentialness and satisfaction, realizing that inside the specialty of deep rooted health lies the significant ability to carry on with a daily existence that twists with wellbeing and delight every step of the way.

11.2 Laying out Sensible Objectives for Enduring Outcomes: Clearing the Way to Feasible Achievement**

In the stupendous embroidery of desires, defining reasonable objectives turns into the lively brushstroke that lays out a representation of accomplishment and satisfaction. Like gifted pilots, we graph a course towards progress, it is deliberate and feasible to guarantee that each step. In this section, we embark on a compelling and engaging journey to learn about the profound impact that setting attainable goals can have on our personal development and success in the long run.

1. Embracing Deliberate Intentions

At the core of defining sensible objectives lies the enabling demonstration of embracing deliberate aims. It is the realization that our objectives are the manifestations of our highest aspirations and desires.

Deliberate goals become the main thrust that moves us forward, adjusting our endeavors to our fantasies.

2. Recognizing Clear and Quantifiable Outcomes

Inside the domain of sensible objective setting, we track down the groundbreaking force of recognizing clear and quantifiable results. We make our progress measurable and trackable by dividing our goals into distinct milestones. Clear and quantifiable results become the compass that keeps us on course.

3. The Soulful Art of Balancing Ambition and Realism
 We discover the soulful art of balancing ambition and realism in the captivating pursuit of long-lasting results. While laying out testing objectives moves development, guaranteeing they are reachable upgrades our inspiration. Offsetting desire with authenticity permits us to extend our cutoff points while keeping pride.

4. Setting Realistic Goals:

The Art of Prioritizing Short-Term and Long-Term Aspirations Prioritizing short-term and long-term goals is an art. Transient objectives give fast wins and force, pushing us towards bigger achievements. Our journey is given direction and a reason to be, and long-term goals encourage transformation.

5. Creating Action Plans

We discover the harmonious rhythm of creating action plans in the symphony of setting realistic goals. An activity plan frames the means and assets expected to accomplish our goals. With a very much created plan, we explore through difficulties and remain fixed on our way to progress.

6. Embracing Adaptability and Adaptability

In the spellbinding domain of enduring outcomes, we track down the endearing notes of embracing adaptability and versatility. Life is dynamic, and conditions might change along our excursion. By staying open to changes, we track down creative ways of conquering snags and remain strong.

7. Tracking Progress and Celebrating Achievements
We discover the transformative power of tracking progress and recognizing accomplishments within the symphony of setting realistic goals. Consistently evaluating our headway keeps us responsible and spurred. Commending every achievement, regardless of how little, builds up our responsibility and lifts our certainty.

8. Gaining from Setbacks

Inside the craft of enduring outcomes lies the insight of gaining from misfortunes. Challenges are inescapable on our way to progress, however they give important illustrations. By thinking about mishaps and involving them as venturing stones, we become smarter and stronger.

Conclusion

A transformative journey of purpose, determination, and development is achieved by setting attainable goals that will yield lasting results. Let each moment serve as an opportunity to appreciate meaningful progress and accomplishments as you pursue your goals. Accept the fact that setting attainable goals is essential to long-term success. Inside the hug of defining reasonable objectives for enduring outcomes lies the way into an existence of satisfaction, progress, and vast self-awareness. Thus, let the core values of deliberate expectations and flexibility lead you towards a universe of supportable accomplishment and satisfaction, realizing that inside the craft of defining reasonable objectives lies the significant ability to make a day to day existence that twists with progress and happiness at each achievement.

11.3 Observing Advancement and Achievement:

Celebrating progress and success emerges as the enchanting melody that elevates our journey and fills it with the sweet notes of joy and fulfillment. Embracing the Art of Joyful Acknowledgment** Like an excellent celebration, we assemble to respect our endeavors, regardless of how large or little, and loll in the gleam of our achievements. In this segment, we set out on a convincing and connecting excursion to investigate the groundbreaking force of praising advancement and achievement, uncovering the significant effect it can have on our inspiration, prosperity, and generally speaking feeling of achievement.

1. Embracing the Art of Gratitude

The empowering act of embracing the art of Gratitude is at the heart of celebrating progress and success. Appreciation turns into the groundwork of our festival, as we express sincere gratitude for the open doors, backing, and gifts that have made ready for our accomplishments. Humility and a profound appreciation for our journey are found in gratitude.

2. Recognizing Big and Small Milestones

Recognizing big and small milestones has the transformative power to celebrate progress and success. Each step in the right direction is a victory by its own doing, and by recognizing our advancement, we track down inspiration to proceed with the excursion towards our objectives. Praising each achievement turns into a festival of our assurance and devotion.

3. Developing a Positive Mindset

In the enamoring quest for cheerful affirmation, we uncover the profound craft of developing a positive outlook. Positive mentality recognizes opportunities and challenges as well as their potential. We build the resilience necessary to overcome future challenges and reinforce our belief in our abilities as we celebrate our progress.

4. Sharing Our Success with Others
The wisdom of sharing our successes with others lies within the art of celebrating progress and success. Our sense of community and connection are bolstered when we celebrate our successes with friends, family, and coworkers. We spread happiness far and wide when we invite others to share in our celebration.

5. Considering Individual Growth

In the orchestra of cheerful affirmation, we find the agreeable mood of pondering self-improvement. Every accomplishment turns into an impression of our development, both in abilities and character. By stopping to reflect, we recognize the changes we have gone through on our excursion.

6. Taking Minutes to Recharge

In the dazzling domain of praising advancement and achievement, we track down the endearing notes of taking minutes to re-energize. Celebrations provide chances to unwind and re energize. By carving out an opportunity to re-energize, we support our spirits and return to our undertakings with recharged energy.

7. Cultivating a Culture of Celebration

Inside the orchestra of blissful affirmation, we uncover the groundbreaking force of encouraging a culture of festivity. Celebrate success and progress as a group in organizations and communities to build bonds and foster a sense of community. A culture of celebration fosters a motivating and upbeat atmosphere.

8. Motivating New Heights

Inside the specialty of commending progress and achievement lies the insight of rousing new levels. Every festival turns into a venturing stone to new desires, rousing us to go after significantly more prominent accomplishments. By celebrating progress, we make a pattern of motivation and strengthening.

Conclusion A transformative journey of joy, gratitude, and motivation can be had by celebrating progress and success. Let each moment serve as an opportunity to practice the art of joyful acknowledgment as you navigate life's milestones. Accept that celebrating progress is not an act of self-indulgence but rather an expression of self-empowerment and appreciation for your efforts. The key to a life of joy, inspiration, and limitless achievement lies within the embrace of celebrating progress and success. Knowing that the profound power to create a life that resonates with fulfillment and contentment at every stage lies within the art of joyful acknowledgment, allows the guiding

principles of gratitude and reflection to lead you toward
a world of celebration and growth.

CONCLUSION

Conclusion: The pursuit of healthy living and lasting fulfillment becomes the vibrant thread that weaves a tale of empowerment, growth, and joy in this grand tapestry of life. Embracing the Journey of Healthy Living and Lasting Fulfillment..We have looked into the transformative power of holistic wellness, set attainable goals, celebrated progress, and developed resilience throughout this journey. Together, these core values form an orchestra that fits our whole self, driving us towards a daily existence that twists with reason and unfathomable prosperity.

As we explore through the parts of our lives, let every second turn into a chance to embrace careful living and cognizant decisions. We have found the significant effect of sustaining sound propensities and looking for proficient help while required, making ready for self-improvement and self-revelation. Resilience enables us to overcome obstacles and embrace adaptability in the face of change with every step we take.

Healthy living is not a destination; rather, it is a lifelong commitment. It expects us to praise our advancement and victories, recognizing every achievement as a demonstration of our assurance and commitment. In the soul of appreciation, we track down lowliness and value the endowments that encompass us.

Let us cultivate a culture of celebration and celebrate each victory as we move with the rhythm of life. A symphony of happiness, support, and inspiration emerges from our collective efforts, reaching far beyond our individual endeavors.

We become stewards of our planet and leave a legacy of abundance and harmony for future generations by pursuing long-term sustainability. We can build a life with meaning and happiness if we recognize the value of rest, food, and healthy relationships.

Let us cultivate compassion and kindness toward ourselves and others on this magical journey toward healthy living and lasting fulfillment. May we generally recall that every misfortune is a chance for development, and each challenge is a venturing stone to win.

Let us carry the guiding principles, a compass that directs us toward a life of vibrant health, meaningful connections, and unwavering contentment, with us as we come to the end of this odyssey. This orchestra of well being and satisfaction is definitely not a solitary note yet an amicable mix of every one of our decisions and activities.

Thus, embrace the excursion of sound living and enduring satisfaction, realizing that inside your heart lies the ability to deeply impact an existence of direction, bliss, and unlimited prosperity. You make a contribution to a symphony that reverberates throughout history with each step you take, leaving behind a legacy of love and inspiration for future generations.

The journey toward healthy living and lasting fulfillment continues to unfold in the grand symphony of life, guided by the melodies of purpose, perseverance, and gratitude. We discover that the pursuit of well-being is a tapestry that weaves together our physical, mental, and emotional experiences as we delve deeper into this wondrous odyssey. As we do so, we uncover new layers of meaning as well as new insights.

As time passes, we embrace the specialty of careful living, tracking down magnificence in the least difficult minutes and loving the present as a gift. We are able to savor the flavors of life, such as the taste of a nourishing meal, the touch of a loved one, or the sight of a breathtaking sunrise, thanks to mindfulness, which becomes our ally.

Chasing enduring outcomes, we figure out how to work out some kind of harmony among desire and authenticity. We set forth towards our objectives with resolute assurance, powered by the information that each step we take is an achievement on our excursion to progress. As we explore the tides of life, we stay versatile, open to change, and anxious to embrace new open doors that current themselves en route.

We take a moment to consider our personal development and transformation in the midst of our endeavors. We witness the development of our strengths and character development with each accomplishment. We are aware that our path is not straight ahead; rather, it is a spiral of growth and learning in which we constantly reach new heights while also spiraling back to incorporate previous lessons.

As we luxuriate in the sparkle of our achievements, we welcome others to participate in our festival, for shared delight enhances our feeling of local area and interconnectedness. We collectively produce a positive and inspiring ripple effect that goes beyond individual achievement.

Beyond the individual, we are aware of our responsibility as planet stewards who are tasked with promoting long-term sustainability. We want to preserve the beauty and resources of our planet for future generations by protecting the environment through conscious choices and collective efforts.

We discover that the sum of our experiences and connections along the way, not the destination, defines our fulfillment on this journey toward healthy living and lasting fulfillment. We embrace the recurring pattern of life, realizing that even notwithstanding difficulties, we have the solidarity to rise, similar to a phoenix from the cinders.

As we finish up this section of our excursion, we anticipate new skylines and unseen experiences, realizing that the quest for prosperity is a deep rooted way, woven into the actual texture of our reality. We join the rhythm of the universe in embracing the symphony of life with every breath we take and every step we take.

So, let's keep going on this amazing journey toward healthy living and lasting happiness by treating each moment as a chance to grow and valuing the connections we make along the way. The key to a life of vibrant health, meaningful purpose, and limitless well-being lies within the embrace of this journey. Let us continue to work together to create a symphony of happiness, perseverance, and love, leaving behind a lasting legacy of hope and fulfillment for the generations to come.

Notepad